An Ethics of Clinical Uncertainty

This book explores the ethical implications of managing uncertainty in clinical decision-making during the COVID-19 pandemic. It develops an ethics of clinical uncertainty that brings together insights from the clinical and biomedical ethical literatures.

The book sets out to recognize the central role uncertainty plays in clinical decision-making and to acknowledge the different levels, kinds, and dimensions of clinical uncertainty. It also aims to aid clinicians and patients in managing clinical uncertainty and to recognize the ethical duty they have to manage clinical uncertainty. The book addresses four ethical duties related to clinical uncertainty: (1) to advance the welfare of those in clinical medicine, (2) to respect the rights of those in clinical medicine, (3) to promote just access to health care, and (4) to care for one another in clinical medicine. These duties took on select urgency during the COVID-19 pandemic because clinical risk assessments about COVID-19 were limited, we were asked to give informed consent in the context of limited and changing knowledge, the pandemic unearthed myriad problems about the distribution of health care, and the pandemic raised questions about how we care for each other in medicine.

An Ethics of Clinical Uncertainty will appeal to scholars, advanced students, and medical professionals working in philosophy of medicine, biomedical ethics, clinical medicine, nursing, public health care, and gerontology.

Mary Ann G. Cutter is currently Professor of Biomedical Ethics in the Department of Philosophy at the University of Colorado at Colorado Springs. She joined the department in 1988 and holds a Ph.D. in Philosophy from Georgetown University through the Kennedy Institute of Ethics Program. She is the author of numerous publications in biomedical ethics, including *The Ethics of Gender-Specific Disease* (Routledge, 2012), *Thinking through Breast Cancer: A Philosophical Exploration of Diagnosis, Treatment, and Survival* (2018), and *Death: A Reader* (2019).

Routledge Annals of Bioethics
Series Editors:
Mark J. Cherry
St. Edward's University, USA
Ana Smith Iltis
Wake Forest University, USA

For more information about this series, please visit: www.routledge.com/Routledge-Annals-of-Bioethics/book-series/RAB

An Ethics of Clinical Uncertainty

Lessons from the COVID-19 Pandemic

Mary Ann G. Cutter

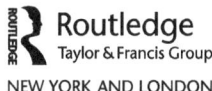

Routledge
Taylor & Francis Group

NEW YORK AND LONDON

First published 2024
by Routledge
605 Third Avenue, New York, NY 10158

and by Routledge
4 Park Square, Milton Park, Abingdon, Oxon, OX14 4RN

Routledge is an imprint of the Taylor & Francis Group, an informa business

ISBN: 978-1-032-62099-2 (hbk)
ISBN: 978-1-032-62098-5 (pbk)
ISBN: 978-1-032-62097-8 (ebk)

DOI: 10.4324/9781032620978

Typeset in Sabon
by Newgen Publishing UK

I dedicate this project to those who have died from COVID-19, those who have suffered from COVID-19, the health care professionals who have worked with COVID-19 patients, and laypersons who have cared for those with COVID-19. These have been heroes in our midst.

Contents

Preface

"Uncertainty is the only certainty we have." (one of those certainties we often hear expressed).

In February 2020, I was drafting a book on managing uncertainty in decision-making in cancer medicine. As a biomedical ethicist and cancer survivor, I have written on breast cancer and wanted to continue my work on the challenges of managing uncertainty in the diagnosis, prognosis, and treatment of breast cancer. As any breast cancer patient or survivor knows, uncertainty marks the terrain of decisions that are made in a field that develops quickly and carries significant practical implications for patients and their families. Despite my best-laid plans in early 2020 when the COVID-19 pandemic hit the U.S., I found myself giving talks on managing clinical uncertainty during the COVID-19 pandemic. In my talks, we tried to come to terms with the uncertainties we all faced as the pandemic spread, our lives changed, and we made decisions under a great deal of uncertainty. Then, in Spring 2022, I taught for the academic organization Semester at Sea and boarded a ship, the *MV World Odyssey*, to teach undergraduate courses in biomedical ethics and the philosophy of death and dying. While teaching on the ship over a four-month period in the Mediterranean and surrounding areas, the shipboard community experienced on a daily basis the challenges of managing uncertainty during the pandemic. Our travels to Italy, Greece, Cyprus, Croatia, Malta, Spain, Gibraltar, Portugal, France, Scotland, Denmark, Sweden, and Germany were preoccupied with different COVID-19 protocols and requirements for entry into different countries, self-assessments and testing for COVID-19, in-country isolation and quarantine practices, and a sundry of other land and sea protocols. Over 104 days, we experienced 8 itinerary changes, 5 days in lockdown on the ship due to a significant rise of COVID-19 cases, and more than 20 COVID-19 tests during our travels, not including the ones we had before and after our time together on the ship. During my class field trips, we visited clinicians in Spain, France, and Scotland to discuss the challenges they experienced during the pandemic. Managing clinical uncertainty emerged as a shared theme. Given these events, my research on clinical uncertainty in the context of cancer care morphed into research about managing clinical uncertainty during a pandemic. And so this project, *An Ethics of Clinical Uncertainty: Lessons from the COVID-19 Pandemic*, took shape.

Acknowledgments

I thank reviewers for their insightful feedback on this project, and for pointing me in the direction of additional readings on the topics raised here. I am grateful to the University of Colorado at Colorado Springs (UCCS) for continued and long-standing support of my work in the philosophy of medicine and biomedical ethics. I am grateful to be part of an organization that has navigated the COVID-19 pandemic thoughtfully, fluidly, and transparently. In particular, I thank my colleagues in the Department of Philosophy at UCCS, and in particular Raphael Sassower, Lorraine Arangno, Sonja Tanner, Jeff Scholes, and Rex Welshon, and my dear friends, Laura Christensen, Mari McGuiness, Raffaela DiBauda, Pete Seel and Kay Collins, Birgit Trauer, and Lisa and Dan Bianca, for being in my COVID-19 "pod" during the pandemic. I thank Semester at Sea, a teaching organization run by Colorado State University, and in particular my Academic Deans Bob Kling and Chris Seng, for giving me an opportunity to travel with 400+ students during Spring 2022 in order to study ethical issues raised during the COVID-19 pandemic. I thank my students who journeyed with me as we figured things out in the classroom, online, and life during the pandemic. In particular, I thank my pre-med student Naila Tagoilelagi for her feedback on this project and the department's research assistant, Tyler Jungbauer, for his assistance in formatting figures. I am so very grateful to my husband, Lewis Cutter, Jr.; my children, Lewis and Paige Cutter, Theresa Cutter, and John Cutter and Christine Nolan; my grandchildren, Sam, Maggie, Ben, Skyler, and Paxton; and Vera Silvestro Gardell for their unconditional support of my academic pursuits and the memories that we have built together during the pandemic. Thankfully, we will move on from the pandemic, and let's hope that the lessons that we have learned about managing clinical uncertainty will remain with us well into the future.

Colorado Springs and Steamboat Springs, Colorado
October 5, 2023

1 Introduction

Focus of Considerations

I write this project on managing uncertainty in clinical decision-making as the global COVID-19 pandemic unfolds across the world and the U.S., and in the state of Colorado. I write this as I am asked to leave my traditional university office and classroom, shelter at home, teach remotely on a full-time basis, voyage with 400+ undergraduate college students on a ship, continue my research and service work, participate in discussions about ethical issues raised by COVID-19, and monitor any personal symptoms I and my loved ones develop. If I have viral symptoms, I am asked to begin making a series of decisions about testing, responses, and recommended interventions. Such decisions are to be made in a world of clinical uncertainty about COVID-19. Over these past few years, the questions have been unending: What is the severe acute respiratory syndrome coronavirus 2 (SARS-CoV-2) and the clinical condition we call COVID-19? Which variants should we be concerned about? How do we know that someone has COVID-19? How can we make sense out of the different symptoms reported by patients? What is "long COVID" and why do some experience this and others do not? How does the virus SARS-CoV-2 cause COVID-19? Does SARS-CoV-2 spread through inhalation, deposition on surfaces, touch, or somehow else? What are the risks of exposing myself to the virus, going to the grocery store, gathering with loved ones, traveling by car or plane, venturing to a doctor's office or health care facility for an annual visit, and going into work? What are the recommended tests for COVID-19? What kind of test (e.g., antigen or PCR) is best? How often should I test for COVID-19? Do the tests detect the variants? If so, how? If not, is this an issue? Are there reliable ways to predict the course of COVID-19? Why were earlier estimates of COVID-19 cases and deaths from COVID-19 so underestimated? Why do some become reinfected with SARS-CoV-2 and others do not? Why do some die from COVID-19 and others do not? What populations are most vulnerable to

DOI: 10.4324/9781032620978-1

COVID-19 and why? What is the best way to treat COVID-19? What populations of patients benefit most from which treatments? What can be done to prevent against COVID-19? What constitutes recommended viral precautions, use of masks and gloves, social (or physical) distancing, quarantines and isolations, and lockdowns? What vaccine works best and how many boosters are recommended or required over what period of time? If I am cautious about getting the vaccine, do I have "vaccine hesitancy"? What constitutes a legitimate reason to refuse the vaccine: medical, governmental, religious, and/or personal? Post being vaccinated, what are the limits on my engagements at home, at work, and in travel? What precautions do I need to follow? Why was it so difficult to distribute medical resources well during the pandemic? Have we sufficiently addressed issues regarding health care inclusion and "disclusion," and ageism and racism, in medicine? What were the reasons for restricting loved ones and allied health care workers (e.g., social workers, pastoral counselors) from seeing patients who were dying from COVID-19? What were the reasons for putting patients who died from COVID-19 in empty closets, unmarked refrigerator trucks, and mass graves? What does a post–COVID-19 world look like? What habits and practices have we acquired that we will want to continue? What habits and practices will we want to eliminate? When will this pandemic be an endemic, a "twindemic" (COVID-19 and the flu), or a "tripledemic" (COVID-19, the flu, and respiratory syncytial virus [RSV])? When will the pandemic be over? Despite all health care professionals know and can do, there has been and remains today much uncertainty about the diagnosis, prognosis, treatment, and prevention of COVID-19.

Responses to these and other questions vary depending on whom one consults at what point in time during the pandemic. Simply put, responses range on a continuum from clear and unequivocal answers to "they just don't know." Responses vary in terms of how individuals process information cognitively, behaviorally, emotionally, socially, economically, and institutionally. They vary in terms of one's experience in making decisions under uncertainty, and how one deals with the unknown, ambiguity, loss of control, and the fears and anxieties that are raised in such situations. They vary in terms of how one deals with risk and the constraints presented in one's own life. They vary in terms of what we have learned and what we have failed to learn about managing clinical uncertainty.

There are insights that can be drawn from these varied responses to COVID-19. Our responses to what we have experienced have set up levels, dimensions, and kinds of clinical uncertainty that patients and their health care providers manage while making decisions. There is uncertainty about what and how we know the clinical condition we call COVID-19. There is uncertainty about the etiology, diagnosis, prognosis, treatment, and prevention of COVID-19. There is uncertainty about the ethical or moral values that arise during a pandemic, those having to do with the welfare and rights of patients and health care professionals, as well as what constitutes just access to health care and how we care for each other in medicine. There is uncertainty about how our systems and institutions have responded to our health care needs during the medical crisis. Further, there are uncertainties about our own uncertainties. After living in a cancer and now COVID-19 world, I now understand what Dr. Osler tells us: "medicine is a science of uncertainty and the art of probability" (Bean, 1950, 125).

Given this, we owe ourselves some time for reflection on how we have managed clinical uncertainty during the COVID-19 pandemic. To begin with, it is important to process what so many of us as patients, clinicians, family members, friends, and members of institutions have experienced during the pandemic. We have witnessed a notable level of clinical uncertainty during the pandemic. We have had to grapple with unprecedented changes in our personal and public lives. We have become a bit more familiar with the realities of disease, illness, dying, and death. We have experienced the limits of medicine and public health measures during a time when we needed a lot from our leaders, health care providers, and institutions. And some, more than others, have experienced unequitable treatment in medicine because of their age, race, ethnicity, and economic status. In light of this inquiry, we find ourselves in need of understanding the role of uncertainty in clinical decision-making. We find ourselves in need of guidance about how to manage clinical uncertainty in the decisions we make in medicine. We need this not simply for how we cognitively process our decisions; we need this for our ethical conscience.

This book explores the ethical implications of managing uncertainty in clinical decision-making during the COVID-19 pandemic. It develops an ethics of clinical uncertainty that brings together insights from the clinical and biomedical ethical literatures. The project has five goals: it sets out (1) to recognize the central role uncertainty plays in clinical decision-making and (2) to map out intersectional levels, kinds, and dimensions of clinical uncertainty. It aims (3) to aid clinicians and patients in managing clinical uncertainty and (4) to recognize the ethical duties clinicians and patients have to manage clinical uncertainty in order to advance the welfare of those in clinical medicine, to respect their rights, to promote justice, and to care for one another in clinical relationships. In the end it offers (5) suggestions for managing moral distress and building moral resilience.

What distinguishes this project are the second and fourth goals. Regarding the second, the project defends an expanded and intersectional account of clinical uncertainty that contrasts with the account typically available in the literature. The account is expanded beyond an epistemological account to include ontological and axiological dimensions.

It is intersectional in that it provides a lens to consider how different identities (e.g., patient and clinician, old and young, privileged and disenfranchised) differentially impact experiences of clinical problems and their care in medicine. Regarding the fourth goal, the project defends the view that managing clinical uncertainty is an ethical duty in clinical medicine. Recognizing an ethical duty to manage clinical uncertainty takes on select urgency during the COVID-19 pandemic. This is because clinical risk assessments about COVID-19 were limited, we were asked to give informed consent in the context of limited and changing knowledge, the pandemic unearthed a myriad of problems about the distribution of health care, and the pandemic raised questions about how we care for each other in medicine.

This project is intended for audiences interested in discussions at the intersection of medicine and philosophy, and medicine and ethics. These include professionals in philosophy of medicine, biomedical ethics, clinical medicine and nursing, public health care, and geriatrics. It also includes health care professionals who have unfinished business to work through after stepping up and serving during the pandemic. The project is intended for patients as well, and for those who seek to reflect on what we just went through during the COVID-19 pandemic and to offer an opportunity to pause, reflect, and debrief. It is intended for those who think about how we might go forward in medicine with some lessons about managing clinical uncertainty, managing moral distress, and building moral resilience. As a member of both groups, a practicing clinical bioethicist and former patient, I find myself in both camps, and so this project can be seen as a product of my own attempt to reflect on lessons from the pandemic. A secondary market comprises informed readers in book clubs interested in how to manage clinical uncertainty when making decisions in medicine. In this way, this project offers both clinical professionals and patients an opportunity to reflect on lessons from the pandemic about managing clinical uncertainty.

To further contextualize, a defining feature of this project is its focus on the ethical implications of managing clinical uncertainty within the context of the clinician–patient relationship. Typically, the clinical literature focuses on the epistemic, or knowledge-based, character of clinical uncertainty. It probes what it means to be uncertain, or doubtful, in one's clinical claims and assumes that clinical nature can be known. Separately, the biomedical ethical literature focuses on moral issues that arise from being uncertain about one's clinical claims or about not being able to act on one's claims because of external or institutional restrictions. This project brings together prominent literature on clinical uncertainty from the clinical and biomedical ethical literature in order to show that both analyses are needed, and they are needed together. It advances an account of "an ethics of clinical uncertainty," thus expanding the discussions on clinical uncertainty and the practice of managing it.

While this project addresses a number of issues, it does not address a host of others. Five issues come to mind. First, the project offers *an* ethics of clinical uncertainty, and not a universal account. Any ethics of clinical uncertainty will need to be developed within the context of particular clinical specialties, and thereby address the particular epistemic, ontological, and evaluative challenges raised therein. Second, the project focuses on the role of clinical uncertainty in the context of making a decision about a clinical course of action in the context of the health care professional–patient relationship. It does not address other contexts, such as making decisions in clinical research, clinical administration, or public health policy and law, although there are implications in those contexts for what is said here. Third, the project draws mainly from discussions of decision-making in the case of the diagnosis, prognosis, treatment, and prevention of COVID-19 between February 2020 and May 2023. It does not focus on what happens before and after this period of the pandemic, although the general lessons here about navigating uncertainty remain applicable well after the pandemic. Fourth, the project focuses on clinical decision-making in the face of uncertainty by competent patients and health care professionals. It does not focus on cases in which the patient or clinician is legally or clinically determined to be incompetent. Fifth, the project focuses primarily on what has occurred in the U.S. and does not address global clinical responses to COVID-19 and the global bioethical issues that arise from them. Nevertheless, the discussion carries implications for managing uncertainty on a global scale in clinical medicine given that there are a number of responses to the pandemic that nations have shared across the globe.

The Case of COVID-19

Let us begin with what we know or think we know about COVID-19 and its diagnosis, prognosis, treatment, and prevention, as of early 2023. For the informed COVID-19 reader, this section can be skipped. For others seeking a brief summary, here is what we think we know. COVID-19, was first reported in China in late 2019 and emerged in the U.S. in mid-March 2020. On February 11, 2020, the World Health Organization officially named it in accordance with conventions adopted by the International Committee on Taxonomy of Viruses (ICTV) (World Health Organization, 2020). It also announced the cause of COVID-19 as the virus SARS-CoV-2. A coronavirus is a large family of different viruses, some of which lead to the common cold, and others of which lead to more serious conditions, such as SARS (severe acute respiratory syndrome), Ebola (a condition brought about by a filovirus, or single-stranded negative-sense RNA virus), and COVID-19 (the clinical condition that currently commands our attention). A coronavirus is named as such because it typically consists of a nucleic acid molecule in a protein host and surrounded by a "corona" or halo ("Coronavirus History," 2020). Although debates remain, SARS-CoV-2 is believed to spread from bats and pangolins to humans in the open markets in Wuhan, China, before spreading around the globe (Timmer, 2020). Another debate concerns whether COVID-19 originated in a laboratory as a result of "gain of function" research, i.e., research that increases the lethality of a virus by splicing a sequence into its genome (Wehner, 2021; Gordon and Strobel, 2023).

The COVID-19 numbers are notable. On August 14, 2021, as I prepared my curriculum for Semester at Sea, there were 36.4 million cases of COVID-19 in the U.S. (Centers for Disease Control, 2021a) and 205.3 million cases in the world (World Health Organization, 2021). There were 617.8 thousand deaths in the U.S. and 4.3 million deaths in the world (Centers for Disease Control, 2021a). On August 14, 2022, and one year later after returning from overseas, there were 92.7 million cases of COVID-19 in the U.S. and 590 million cases in the world. There were 1.03 million deaths in the U.S. and 6.4 million deaths in the world (Centers for Disease Control, 2022a). For another perspective on numbers, and in December 2020 in the U.S. during the Delta outbreak and before the availability of vaccines, there was a 43% increase in deaths overall. In January 2022 during the Omicron outbreak and after the availability of vaccines, there was a 37% increase in deaths overall (Hutto, 2022). In 2023, while the number of deaths from or with COVID-19 is going down, many continue to struggle with the effects of the viral infection.

Consider that individuals from particular populations (e.g., the elderly; members of racial, ethnic, or economic groups; the uninsured; males) are more likely to contract COVID-19, be quite sick from it, and die from it. As Meredith Freed and her colleagues at the Kaiser Family Foundation report,

> [a]s of the week ending October 1, 2022, the United States has lost nearly 1.1 million lives to COVID-19, of which about 790,000 are people ages 65 and older. People 65 and older account for 16% of the total US population but 75% of all COVID deaths to date.
>
> (2022)

Further, Black, Hispanic, AIAN (Alaskan Native), and NHOPI (Native Hawaiian and Other Pacific Islander) people have been more likely to contract COVID-19 and suffer debilitating consequences. As Latoya Hill and Samantha Artiga report,

[a]s of August 5, 2022, the Centers for Disease Control and Prevention (CDC) reported a total of over 84 million cases, for which race/ethnicity was known for 65% or over 55 million, and a total of over 880,000 deaths, for which race/ethnicity was known for 85% or over 750,000.

(2022)

Still further, individuals who lacked insurance were more vulnerable to COVID-19. As Stan Dorn and Rebecca Gordan report,

[n]ationally, roughly 1 out of every 3 COVID-19 deaths are linked to health insurance gaps. More than 40% of all COVID-19 infections are associated with health insurance gaps. By August 31, 2020, health insurance gaps were linked to an estimated 2.6 million COVID-19 cases and 58,000 COVID-19 deaths. By February 1, 2021, 10.9 million infections and 143,000 COVID-19 deaths may have been associated with health insurance gaps.

(2021)

In terms of sex differences in sequelae from COVID-19 infection, and early in the pandemic,

it was noted that the severity of acute illness, rates of intensive care admission, and COVID-19 related mortality were greater among male patients than female patients, whereas the opposite tread was observed with long COVID syndrome, where females are more affected.

(Sylvester et al., 2022)

Clinically speaking, COVID-19 involves a significant respiratory illness with symptoms, such as fever or chills, coughing, shortness of breath or difficulty breathing, fatigue, muscle or body aches, headache, loss of taste or smell, sore throat, congestion or runny nose, nausea or vomiting, and/or diarrhea (Centers for Disease Control, 2022d), depending on the variant and one's immunization status. Serious cases of COVID-19 are marked by an acute respiratory infection, a blood response, and an intense cytokine immunological reaction, which results in a marked inflammatory response that can be painful, challenging to treat, and deadly.

The diagnosis of COVID-19 starts with taking into consideration the signs and symptoms of the presenting patient, and in particular those of the respiratory tract. Symptomatic patients are tested for SARS-CoV-2 using nucleic acid amplification testing (NAAT), and most commonly the reverse-transcription polymerase chain reaction (RT-PCR) assay. In widespread public testing, the antigen test is an acceptable alternative because it is easier to administer, but sensitivity is lower than with NAATs.

Vaccination status does not influence the interpretation of the vital test results. As of this writing, both the PCR and antigen tests detect the viral variants, including Omicron (Caliendo and Hanson, 2022).

If one thinks about it, COVID-19 is not one disease condition. COVID-19 constitutes a cluster of clinical conditions brought about by variants or mutations of SARS-CoV-2 and treated by specialists from infectious disease, immunology, and neurology, among others. Here, a variant is a viral genome or genetic code that contains one or more mutations. In August 2021, there were a large number of variants, including Alpha, Beta, Gamma, Delta, Eta, Lota, Kappa, and Lamda. As we all well know, one of the variants that was particularly contagious in July 2021 in the U.S. was the Delta variant, which according to the World Health Organization caused 80% to 87% of all COVID-19 cases during the last two weeks of July 2021 (World Health Organization, 2022). The Delta variant of COVID-19 was quite severe for those over 65 years old and those with comorbidities, leading to a significant rise in hospitalizations that challenged urban and rural hospital capacities (Centers for Disease Control, 2021d). And then things changed. During the first two weeks of January 2022, more than 90% of COVID-19 cases resulted from the Omicron variants of COVID-19 (Centers for Disease Control, 2022c). Compared to Delta, Omicron was more contagious, less virulent or severe, and spread in 48–72 hours, as opposed to the 7–10 days. As of this writing, additional variants (e.g., BA.2.86) have emerged, as one would expect with any virus.

In order to establish a sense of transmissibility and severity of the virus, the World Health Organization classified the SARS-CoV-2 variants as follows: "variants of concern" (VOCs; e.g., Delta, Omicron, and their variants) and "variants of interest" (VOIs; e.g., Alpha, Beta, and Gamma, and their subsets). Here, VOCs have been the ones to watch. They refer to those that demonstrate one or more of the following changes "at a degree of global public health significance":

- Increase in transmissibility or detrimental change in COVID-19 epidemiology; OR
- Increase in virulence or change in clinical disease presentations; OR
- Decrease in effectiveness of public health and social measures or available diagnostics, vaccines, and therapeutics (World Health Organization, 2022).

Alternatively, VOIs refer to those variants that are being monitored and do not yet rise to the level of VOCs. The determination of such classifications reflects the ease of viral spread, the associated disease severity, and the performance of vaccines, therapeutic medicines, diagnostic tools, and other public health and social measures. Here we see that clinical nosologies (i.e., classifications) and nosographies (i.e., descriptions) are not simply about the facts of a biological entity, but include evaluations of how best to respond to it. More on this will be said in Chapter 4.

As of this writing, health care professionals are monitoring what is called "long COVID," "long COVID syndrome," "long-haul COVID," "chronic COVID," "Post Acute SARS-CoV-2 Infection," or "Post-COVID Conditions." According to Sylvester et al. (2022), the likelihood of having long COVID is significantly greater among females as opposed to male patients. Long COVID is a heterogeneous phenotypical and neurologic condition characterized by long-lasting symptoms, often of one or so kind (e.g., headaches, joint pain), that go away and come back. Its cause is unknown and there is no diagnosis. Long COVID can entail extreme fatigue, respiratory and heart issues, autoimmune responses, neurological symptoms (e.g., "COVID brain"), pain, and menstrual changes. Its risk factors include severe COVID-19 symptoms, hospitalization, comorbidities or underlying health considerations, and an unvaccinated state. As of this writing, there is no specific treatment, but significant efforts are being made to understand this heterogeneous clinical phenomenon (Centers for Disease Control, 2022c).

Regarding the prognosis of COVID-19, 80% of patients have mild symptoms with full recovery, while 20% of patients develop much more serious disease, such as pneumonia and acute respiratory distress syndrome (ARDS), or acute respiratory distress syndrome (Schleicher et al., 2020).

> For critically ill patients with COVID-19, the prognosis is poor with mortality ranging from 25 to 50 percent that is largely driven by severe ARDS. However, death can occur from several other conditions including cardiac arrhythmia, cardiac arrest, and pulmonary embolism. The highest rates occur in those ≥64 years.
>
> (Anesi, 2022, 13; also see Higgins-Dunn, 2021)

As the pandemic develops, mortality rates have decreased, but length of stay in the hospital has increased, especially for those with comorbidities. Nevertheless, it has been challenging to predict outbreaks of COVID-19 and hospitals have been overwhelmed at times with finding beds and care for patients. Some of this has to do with the sheer volume of patients and some has to do with the so-called Great Resignation, the exodus of workers who faced stress, dissatisfaction with work, or burnout during the pandemic (Linzer et al., 2022). Henry (2022) reports that one out of five physicians report that they plan on leaving clinical practice soon than later given their experience during the pandemic.

Regarding treatment for adults with COVID-19, "[m]any patients with known or suspected COVID-19 have mild disease that does not warrant hospital-level care" (Kim and Ghandi, 2022, 27). Such patients are typically advised to return home and rest, wear a mask when in the company of loved ones, and isolate for 5–10 days, depending on the variant and the recommended protocol. Specific therapy for COVID-19 is generally not recommended for symptomatic individuals without any risk factors for progression to severe disease or individuals who have asymptomatic SARS-CoV-2 infection (Cohen and Gebo, 2022, 3).

Those hospitalized are those with more severe cases of COVID-19, organ dysfunction, or other comorbidities that could complicate potential therapy. Patients hospitalized with COVID-19 are typically given pharmacologic prophylaxis for venus thromboembolism. Acetaminophen is preferred to be used for fever. For patients "who have clinical or laboratory risk factors for severe disease and were hospitalized for COVID-19," remdesivir is advised (Kim and Ghandi, 2022, 28). For COVID-19 patients who are hospitalized for other conditions, therapies such as nirmatrelvir-ritonavir (Paxlovid) or monoclonal antibodies are recommended. For patients with severe oxygen needs, dexamethasone, baricitinib, or tocacilizumab are recommended (Kim and Ghandi, 2022, 29). In 2021, while hydroxychloroquine and chloroquine were recommended under an emergency use authorization, their uses were revoked because both drugs were shown not to be as effective as initially thought. Note as well that some monoclonal-antibody treatments are no longer recommended because they are not effective in targeting the newer variants and subvariants of COVID-19.

For children with mild cases of COVID-19, hospitalization is not required and supportive care at home is recommended. "Indications for hospitalization in children with COVID-19 include: severe or lower respiratory tract disease, nonsevere disease with underlying conditions that increase the risk of severe disease (e.g., immune compromise), and fever in infants younger than 30 days" (Deville et al., 2022, 3). Those with severe or critical disease generally require hospitalization, supportive care (e.g., respiratory support, fluid and electrolyte support, antibiotics, thromboprophylaxis), and ventilatory support, depending on the severity of their condition. Antiviral agents are "considered on a case-by-case basis and preferably occur in the context of a clinical trial" (Deville et al., 2022, 35).

Regarding prevention, in December 2020, the U.S. authorized the use of vaccines for COVID-19. As the U.S. Food and Drug Administration reports, "[t]he Food and Drug Administration (FDA) issued Emergency Use Authorization (EUA) for the Pfizer-BioNTech COVID-19 vaccine on December 11, 2020, and for the Moderna COVID-19 vaccine on December 18, 2020; each is administered as a 2-dose series" (U.S. Food and Drug

Administration, 2021a). In April 2021, the Centers for Disease Control and the Food and Drug Administration "recommended a pause in the use of the Janssen (Johnson & Johnson) COVID-19 vaccine in the United States out of an abundance of caution, effective Tuesday, April 13" (Centers for Disease Control, 2021c). They justified the pause based on the following reason: "Of the 6.8 million Janssen COVID-19 vaccine doses administered in the United States to date, six cases of a type of blood clot called 'cerebral venous sinus thrombosis' (CVST) were seen in combination with low levels of blood platelets (thrombocytopenia)" (Centers for Disease Control, 2021c). On April 23, 2021, the Centers for Disease Control and the Food and Drug Administration lifted the pause (U.S. Food and Drug Administration, 2021b) and the Janssen vaccine became an option along with Pfizer and Moderna in the U.S. health care delivery system.

In late summer 2021, discussions regarding mandatory boosters for COVID-19 emerged. In August 2021, the U.S. recommended that those over 18 years of age get a booster shot eight months after the second shot. A date of September 20, 2021, was announced to have boosters available, and vaccines were slowly rolled out (Centers for Disease Control, 2021c). Subsequently, there were discussions about the timeline between shots (six or eight months), how many boosters were clinically advised (one, two, or more), whether one vaccine was better than the other (depending on the variant), and whether vaccines produced by different manufacturers could be given in sequence. In terms of public attention and debate, the topic of COVID-19 vaccines and boosters has garnered significant attention and discussion these past few years (Preeti et al., 2021).

As of November 2022, the Centers for Disease Control recommended the following with regard to protecting oneself:

To help protect oneself and others from COVID-19:

Get vaccinated and stay up to date on your COVID-19 vaccines.
Everyone ages 2 years and older should properly wear a well-fitting mask indoors in public in areas where the COVID-19 Community Level is high, regardless of vaccination status.
Avoid poorly ventilated spaces and crowds.
Test to prevent spread to others.
Wash your hands often. If soap and water are not readily available, use a hand sanitizer that contains at least 60% alcohol.
Cover coughs and sneezes.
Clean high touch surfaces regularly or as needed and after you have visitors in your home. If someone is sick or has tested positive for COVID-19, disinfect frequently touched surfaces.
Monitor your health daily.

(Centers for Disease Control, 2022b)

If one has possible or confirmed COVID-19:

Stay home except to get medical care.
Monitor your symptoms.
Get tested as soon as possible after your symptoms start.
Get rest and stay hydrated. Take over-the-counter medicines, such as acetaminophen, to help you feel better.
Call ahead before visiting your doctor.
If you are sick, wear a well-fitting mask.

(Centers for Disease Control, 2022b)

On January 30, 2023, the Biden administration announced that the Public Health Emergency (PHE) declaration under Section 319 of the Public Health Service (PHS) Act would expire on May 11, 2023. In early 2023 in the U.S., and since the peak of the Omicron surge at the end of January 2022, daily COVID-19 reported cases decreased by 92%, COVID-19 deaths declined by over 80%, and new COVID-19 hospitalizations were down nearly 80% (U.S. Department of Health and Human Services, 2023). After May 11, 2023, access to COVID-19 vaccines and boosters would still be available, as would treatments such as Paxlovid and Lagevrio.

While most of us would like to put the pandemic behind us as we get back to "normal," we continue to grapple with the effects of COVID-19 in our personal and public lives. Masking is still advised in many institutional settings, our loved ones are still getting sick and some have died from or with COVID-19, health care professionals continue to report significant levels of stress and burnout in the workplace, and we have lost a level of confidence in health care after witnessing its limitations. Some of us have moved on, some of us cannot, but all of us have some opinion about clinical actions during the pandemic. I suggest that one of the underlying challenges during the pandemic that challenged us was managing clinical uncertainty. This project has much to say about that experience.

Outline of Inquiry

This book is divided into nine chapters, including this one, the Introduction. Chapter 1, the Introduction, has set the stage for discussion in this project. Chapter 2 reviews background literature on clinical decision-making and locates this discussion of clinical uncertainty in the quest for certainty. Chapter 3 reviews epistemic definitions of clinical uncertainty found in the clinical literature in terms of three dimensions, source, issue, and locus. Chapter 4 offers an overview of conceptual roots of clinical uncertainty from philosophy of medicine in order to offer a broader interpretation of clinical uncertainty in terms of ontological and axiological considerations.

Ontologically speaking, clinical uncertainty arises from the limits, changes, and complexity of a clinical phenomenon. Axiologically speaking, clinical certainty arises from the values that frame clinical knowledge and nature. Such values are ambiguous, varied, and chosen. Building on Chapters 3 and 4, Chapter 5 offers an expanded and intersectional taxonomy of clinical uncertainty in terms of epistemological, ontological and axiological levels, kinds, and dimensions. Chapter 6 provides suggestions about how to manage clinical uncertainty in light of the broader focus offered in Chapter 5. Chapter 7 explores the ethical or moral duties clinicians and patients have to address clinical uncertainty in order to promote the ethical duties to advance welfare, to respect rights, to promote health equity, and to care for one another in clinical relationships. Chapter 8 explores the challenge of managing moral distress and building moral resilience in medicine in the context of managing clinical uncertainty. Chapter 9 brings the project to a close with a call for "an ethics of clinical uncertainty" and suggestions for future avenues of study.

In the end, the message is this: clinicians and patients have an ethical duty to manage clinical uncertainty. Uncertainty characterizes our knowledge about clinical problems, the nature of clinical problems, and how we value and disvalue them. Managing clinical uncertainty carries significant ethical implications for how welfare is advanced, rights are respected, justice is promoted, and care is practiced in medicine. More specifically, it carries ethical implications for how we manage clinical risks, secure informed consent, promote access to health care, and care for the vulnerable. Managing clinical uncertainty carries significant implications for how we manage moral distress and build moral resilience. While the project focuses on COVID-19, it is not just about COVID-19. It is about managing clinical uncertainty well after the COVID-19 pandemic because clinical uncertainty frames clinical knowledge, clinical problems, and the values that guide actions in medicine.

2 Decision-Making in Clinical Medicine

The Context of Clinical Uncertainty: Clinical Decision-Making

Clinical uncertainty arises in the context of making clinical decisions. Patients make decisions about their health care, choose to seek the attention of health care providers, and health care providers choose a range of options as they diagnose, assess, and manage what patients bring into the clinic. During the COVID-19 pandemic, patients with particular signs and symptoms sought the attention of health care professionals, made decisions about the risks of COVID-19, and consented to or declined tests, treatments, and preventions that clinicians recommended. Clinicians ordered available COVID-19 tests, estimated a patient's prognosis, and recommended available options for interventions. They rallied to find resources and allocated them in accordance with accepted clinical and ethical standards. In these distinct, yet overlapping actions in medicine, patients and clinicians sought to make decisions within the context of limited information, accepted protocol, available resources, and accepted ethical standards.

Granted, there are significant differences in the levels, kinds, and dimensions of clinical uncertainty experienced by clinicians and patients. Clinicians rely on clinical evidence seen through the frames of their clinical training and the values of their profession as they navigate the diagnosis, prognosis, treatment, and prevention of a clinical problem. Patients rely on evidence clinicians provide, supplemented by their own readings and conversations with friends, and make judgments about such evidence within the context of their personal lives. Nevertheless, both clinicians and patients manage the uncertainties raised by knowing and valuing a clinical problem. They do this individually as well as collectively within the clinician–patient relationship. More is said about this in the pages to come.

Returning to the topic at hand, let's spend a bit of time on clinical decision-making. Clinical decision-making is understood as a process in which data is gathered, interpreted, and evaluated within specific contexts

DOI: 10.4324/9781032620978-2

and with regard to a body of data in order to determine an evidence-based course of action (Banning, 2008). As physician Alvan Feinstein says,

> clinical judgment [or decision-making] has a distinctive methodology for dealing with the tangible data of human illness; and clinical judgment now—uniquely in medical history—has both the obligation and the opportunity to be accomplished with scientific taste, discretion, and quality.
>
> (1967, 8)

This chapter considers prominent approaches in clinical decision-making and locates this discussion of clinical uncertainty in a quest for certainty. It reviews three approaches in clinical decision-making, namely, pattern recognition, causal analysis, and probabilistic analysis. Each has historical and conceptual significance in its attempt to classify and describe clinical problems. Each seeks to provide certainty in the diagnosis, prognosis, treatment, and prevention of clinical problems. But medical methodology does not guarantee certainty. A consideration of approaches in clinical decision-making gives us insight into some of the sources of clinical uncertainty and our obligations to manage clinical uncertainty, both topics of which are developed in subsequent chapters.

Approaches in Clinical Decision-Making and the Search for Clinical Certainty

Literature on clinical decision-making provides accounts of how clinicians and patients make decisions in the health care professional–patient relationship (also see Feinstein, 1967; Wulff, 1981; Groopman, 2007; Sox et al., 2013; Hunink, 2014; Vordermark, 2019). These descriptive and prescriptive approaches range from ones that are highly focused on decisions about the biological basis of the disease to ones focused on the care of the patient as a biological, psychological, and social agent (Engel, 1980, 1981). Some of the accounts draw from brain science (Gold and Shadlen, 2007) and others rely on information processing (Berner, 2007), psychological (Barbey et al., 2014), or behavioral economic (Kahneman et al., 1982; Kahneman, 2011) models of clinical decision-making. As one would expect, these accounts cannot fully be separated given that decision-makers are cognitive, psychological, social, and moral agents.

Let's begin our consideration of clinical decision-making by considering three kinds of clinical decision-making approaches found in the clinical literature (Wulff, 1981, 80). These include pattern recognition, causal analysis, and probabilistic analysis. What follows is an oversimplification of decision-making approaches that serve as a basis for getting us started thinking about the role of uncertainty in clinical decision-making. To begin with, *pattern recognition* in clinical decision-making focuses on finding patterns or similarities among clinical problems that present in the clinic (Wulff, 1981, 81). In this case, a pattern is a cluster of signs and symptoms that come together and serve as a basis for the claims that a patient has a particular disease or illness. Here, a typical scenario is that a sick person brings complaints about certain signs and symptoms to the attention of the clinician, and a clinician organizes and distinguishes among such expressions in order to arrive at patterns that fit or do not fit current descriptions and classifications of clinical problems.

Pattern analysis in clinical medicine has a long history. It is rooted in traditional ways of diagnosing patients well before the availability of advanced technology in medicine. In *Nosologia Methodica*, physician François Boissier de Sauvages (1706–1767) offers a taxonomy of disease in terms of ten kinds in terms of what can be observed and documented about a clinical problem:

I.   vitia: injuries of the skin, e.g., punctures
II.   febres: fevers, e.g., influenza
III.   phlegmasiae: inflammations, e.g., smallpox
IV.   spasmi: convulsive diseases, e.g., epilepsy
V.   anhelationes: respiratory disturbances, e.g., asthma
VI.   debilitates: weaknesses, e.g., fainting
VII.   dolores: pains, e.g., heartburn
VIII. vesaniae: mental disturbances, e.g., delirium
IX.   fluxus: discharge of bodily fluids, e.g., diarrhea
X.   cachexiae: physical wasting and deprivation, e.g., leprosy
             (Sauvages, 1768, 92–95; also see, Cutter, 2003, 36).

Sauvages, along with physicians Thomas Sydenham (1624–1689) and William Cullen (1710–1790), sought to organize disease categories in terms of signs and symptoms for purposes of developing treatment warrants. Taken by itself, this way of classifying diseases based on signs and symptoms may seem odd or oversimplified by today's standards, but it marks a notable move in medicine to provide an evidence-based way to understand and treat disease, as opposed to speculative ways of classifying disease. As an example: while classifying fevers (II above) as a disease is fraught with problems of overgeneralizations and lack of specificity for what affects the patient, such an approach is an important step in the development of evolving knowledge about a disease. It focuses on a clinician's *observations* of a patient's signs and symptoms as a basis for understanding and treating them. Such observations are empirical and thereby open to testimony by other observers. Such observations contrast with speculative ways of classifying fever in terms of possession by meta-physical forces.

In the case of COVID-19, consider the following case: A person with a fever of 101 degrees, cough, sore throat, body aches, and difficulty breathing seeks the advice of a health care professional. In turn, the health care professional looks for patterns in what is being expressed and compares patterns found in similar populations and recommends a certain course of testing for COVID-19. If positive with a mild case of COVID-19, the health care professional recommends to the patient a certain course of treatment, such as to return home and rest, wear a mask when in the company of others, and isolate for a recommended number of days. If positive with a serious case of COVID-19, the health care professional recommends that the patient be hospitalized and treated, especially if the signs and symptoms are severe and the patient is over the age of 65 and/or has comorbidities. If negative, the health care professional may recommend that the patient return home and take some over-the-counter medications to treat the symptoms, along with social distancing practices accepted at the time to ward off the spread of the virus.

As an empirical approach to disease, pattern recognition in clinical medicine plays an important role in the determination of what is considered a clinical problem. As physician-philosopher H. Tristram Engelhardt, Jr., says, "[p]atient problems came to be understood as *bona fide* [real or genuine] problems only if they had a pathoanatomical or pathophysiological truth value" (1996, 216). That is, a problem brought to the attention of health care professionals becomes a clinical problem when evidence can be established for it by multiple clinical observers. As Englehardt says, "Absent a lesion or a physiological disturbance to account for the complaint, the complaint was likely to be regarded as *male fide* [not real or genuine]" (1996, 216) in medicine. What distinguishes medicine from, say, biology or law, is the role it plays in addressing patient signs and symptoms for purposes of alleviating the pain and suffering that accompanies disability, deformity, and dysfunction.

A second approach in clinical decision-making is based on an *etiological or causal determination* (Wulff, 1981, 81). An etiological determination in medicine emerges in the seventeenth century with the thinking of philosopher and scientist Francis Bacon (1561–1626) (1878). It includes the statement of a problem, hypothesis formation, collection and analysis of data, and confirmation or rejection of hypothesis geared toward understanding the *relation* between events in nature. A central relation here is causation, the event in which something brings something else about or the relation between cause and effect. In medicine, causation, or etiology as medicine likes to call it, seeks to identify and understand a clinical problem in terms of its cause. Isolating such cause-and-effect relations enables a clinical problem to be explained, predicted, and managed. For instance, establishing that X causes Y disease allows medicine to explain a clinical problem in terms of how it has come about, predict what might occur based on how it has come about, and manage it in terms of its nature, severity, and progression.

Simply put, three kinds of causal relations can be distinguished: necessary, sufficient, and contributory. Necessary causation occurs when B does not occur without A. As an example, SARS-CoV-2 is a necessary condition for COVID-19. Sufficient causation occurs when B always occurs when A does. As an example, SARS-CoV-2 may not be sufficient for COVID-19 because one can be positive for the virus, but not have any symptoms for the clinical problem. Contributory causation occurs when B may or may not occur with A, but there is evidence that it contributes to the clinical problem. As an example, it is unclear what conditions contribute to "long COVID," but we might expect that medicine will provide some explanations in the future in terms of how the clinical problem comes about. Understanding these causal relations allows clinicians to diagnose, predict, treat, and prevent COVID-19.

The move from sign- and symptom-based descriptions and classifications to etiological accounts of a clinical problem is made possible by evidence, a causal way of thinking about clinical problems, and the available technology that can establish such an understanding at a level that is specific and reliable. The early nineteenth century brings about a shift in how, for instance, fever is not a disease, as depicted in Sauvage's clinical taxonomy, but rather a sign or symptom of a condition found in organs, tissue, or cells (Engelhardt, 1996, Ch. 5). For pathologists Robert Koch (1843–1910) and Louis Pasteur (1822–1895), who inaugurated a "germ theory" of disease, fever is a sign or symptom in patients with tuberculosis, and mycobacterium tuberculosis is the etiological agent that causes the bacterial infection called tuberculosis (Honigsbaum, 2019, 6–7). Tuberculosis can in turn be distinguished from streptococcal pneumonia, a bacterial infection caused by streptococcus that inflames the air sacs in the lungs, which in turn is treated differently.

In the case of COVID-19, consider an oversimplified case in which a nursing home patient is transferred to a hospital and presents with a fever of 101 degrees and a productive cough or severe body aches. Here, a clinician observes the patient, takes a medical history, and records the patient's vital signs. The clinician may hypothesize that the patient has COVID-19, not because there is a fever, which is a symptom, but rather because of the presence of a viral agent that brings about the fever. A clinician orders tests, such as a molecular or antigen test for COVID-19, the former of which detects COVID-19's viral RNA and the latter of which detects specific proteins on the surface of COVID-19. A clinician then orders a chest X-ray in order to confirm or reject the hypothesis. If a COVID-19 test comes back negative and the chest X-ray comes back positive for a lower lobe infiltrate (e.g., pus, blood, or protein), the clinician can confirm that the diagnosis is pneumonia and not COVID-19. Such a diagnosis is, of course, not based solely on a single clinician's observation; it is based on the observations of a *community* of clinicians and researchers who have documented such cases and passed those down in conference presentation, peer-reviewed research publications, and clinical protocols. Such observations, research, and protocols remain open to revision and reconsideration based on subsequent observations and research as new knowledge, new medical technology, and new practices and treatments develop and evolve that enhance patient welfare and decrease pain and suffering.

The move from a pattern analysis to an etiological one is important in medicine because it generates new understandings of clinical problems that in turn guide new ways to treat and prevent them (Engelhardt, 1996, Ch. 5). Note that in the move from documenting patient complaints to developing etiological accounts, clinical descriptions and classifications change. In this change, previously unrelated clinical conditions, such as tuberculosis and pneumonia, are seen to be related in terms of a bacterial infection that affects the lungs, but are separable in terms of being brought about by different bacterial agents. Similarly, clinical conditions, such as the common cold and COVID-19, are seen to be related in terms of their being coronaviruses, and similar coronaviruses, such as SARS-CoV (identified in 2003) and SARS-CoV-2 (identified in 2019 and officially named in 2020), are separated in terms of types of coronaviruses that bring about the clinical problem. SARS, for instance, has been treated with supportive care, tracheal intubation, airway management, mechanical ventilation, and/or oxygen therapy (Caldaria et al., 2020). SARS-CoV-2 is treated similarly, and has been the target of additional treatments, including nirmatrelvir/ritonavir (Paxlovid) and molnupira (Cohen and Gebo, 2022).

A third approach in clinical decision-making is a *probabilistic analysis* (Wulff, 1981, 80ff). A probabilistic analysis specifies the extent to which something is likely to occur using quantitative data (Burger and Starbird, 2005). Probability is determined in mathematics by the ratio of the favorable cases to the whole number of cases. It refers to the extent to which something will happen based on a reference population. For instance, consider the statement we often heard in 2020 about COVID-19: "Although more than 80% of patients with COVID-19 infection have mild disease and make a full recovery, a significant proportion of patients progress to pneumonia, and half of these cases will develop severe acute respiratory syndrome (ARDS)" (Schleicher et al., 2020). This means that eight out of ten who test positive for COVID-19 have a mild case of COVID-19 and do not need to be hospitalized. Two out of ten have a more serious case of

COVID-19 and one out of ten will develop ARDS. A probability analysis gives meaningful quantitative value to the occurrence of an outcome or set of events based on a reference population.

A probabilistic analysis in science emerged in the seventeenth century with mathematician and attorney Pierre Fermet (1601–1665) ("Pierre," 2021) and mathematician and philosopher Blaise Pascal (1623–1662) in the context of studying gambling or calculations of probabilities (Todhunter, 1865; Sassower and Grodin, 1987). Regarding calculations of probabilities, the uncertainty of the gain is proportional to the certainty of the stake according to the proportion of the chances of gain and loss. This means that the riskier the action, the more one might want to establish the specific harms that might occur and the less one is inclined to accept a loss. Alternatively, the less riskier the action, the less one might want to establish the specific harms that will occur and the more one might be willing to accept a loss. The

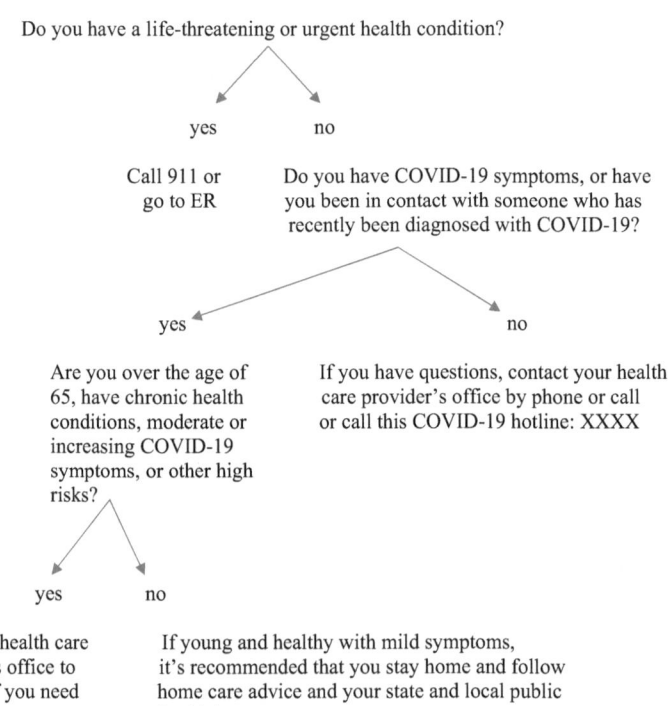

Figure 2.1 Clinical decision tree.

point is that a probabilistic analysis provides a quantitative and qualitative description of how likely an event is to occur in a population.

In the case of COVID-19, consider the following example of a probabilistic decision tree found on websites and in newspapers during the pandemic (see Figure 2.1). This type of decision tree appeared in newspapers across the U.S. during the pandemic. While it does not entail probability values, we can assume that public health officials designed it with probabilities in mind.

As seen here, a probabilistic analysis of a clinical problem provides an account of risk, where risk is the probability of gain or benefit in relation to loss or injury. It relies on pattern analysis of a clinical problem, a causal account of what brings the clinical problem about, and estimates of benefits and loss. Whether the account is simple, as illustrated above, or more sophisticated as found in decision trees that entail statistical data drawn from risk assessment research, a probabilistic analysis differs from a pattern recognition and causal analysis approach in that it provides estimates of the multiple factors contributing to the expression of a clinical problem, In Figure 2.1, for instance, while being exposed to SARS-CoV-2 is necessary, comorbidities such as compromised lung function contribute to the severity of COVID-19, thus providing a more complex account of COVID-19.

Contemporary clinicians and patients rely on a variety of approaches in making decisions in clinical medicine. Physician Donald Woolever provides a helpful overview of the components of clinical decision-making that appeal to pattern recognition, etiological determination, and probabilistic analysis. His summary follows:

1. Determine your *probabilities*. In other words, what is the likelihood that your patient has a specific diagnosis, based on his or her symptoms, history, etc.?
2. Gather data by further evaluating the patient—*additional history, vital signs and physical exam.*
3. *Update your probabilities*, including the pre-test probability of any test you may want to order. Then, carefully, collect and interpret additional data from diagnostic tests.
4. Consider an intervention to see whether it crosses your *treatment threshold* [i.e., in which the treatment has marked benefit for the diseased patient and low risk for the non-diseased patient]. If it does, consider the patient's context before moving forward. If you don't have enough information to convince yourself to cross the threshold, consider other options, which may include gathering additional data or watchful waiting.

(Woolever, 2008, 35, my italics)

In the case of COVID-19, a clinician will:

1 *Determine the probabilities that a patient has COVID-19.* A clinician determines the extent to which the patient presents with a fever of 100 degrees or over OR is feeling feverish AND has one or more symptoms such as a cough, sore throat or body aches, difficulty breathing, fatigue, and a runny or stuffy nose. A clinician takes into consideration the age of the patient, whether the patient has recently traveled and/or has had contact with someone who has been diagnosed with COVID-19, and whether the patient has comorbidities (e.g., diabetes, obesity, respiratory, or heart problems).
2 *Gather additional history, signs, and symptoms by further evaluating the patient.* Depending on what is available, examine the patient to confirm temperature, oxygen flow, lung function, heart function, weight, results from COVID-19 tests, etc.
3 *Update the probabilities that the patient has COVID-19* based on current evidence.
4 *Consider an intervention* if patient reporting, clinical observations, and testing confirm or do not rule out COVID-19. The choices here are to recommend that the patient return home to quarantine with symptomatic treatments such as anti-inflammatory drugs, be admitted to the hospital for observation and more extensive treatment (e.g., antiviral, anti-replication, or anti-inflammatory drugs), targeted toward the signs and symptoms, or be admitted to an ICU for more advanced intervention. Given the accepted clinical standards, a clinician recommends treatments that have been shown to be effective for COVID-19.

As seen here, approaches in clinical decision-making draw on pattern recognition, etiological analysis, and probabilistic analysis. Pattern analysis focuses on bringing organization to the signs and symptoms that bring patients to the attention of health care professionals. Etiological analysis focuses on that which brings a clinical condition about for purposes of treating and preventing it. Probabilistic analysis focuses on the multiple risk factors that play a role in a clinical condition. These approaches require input from clinicians as well as patients for them to be successful. As a consequence, according to Woolever, a *shared decision-making model* captures best how clinicians and patients make decisions in medicine.

The best decisions are often made in partnership with our patients. We have knowledge of diagnostic techniques, diseases, prognoses, treatment options, preventive strategies and the like. Our patients are experts as well. They have knowledge of their prior illnesses, social circumstances, habits and behaviors, risk tolerance, values and preferences.

The process of sharing these two bodies of knowledge has several names, including patient-centered care and informed decision making. I like this definition: the process of interacting with patients to arrive at an informed, values-based choice among medically reasonable alternatives. Of course, not all patients are interested in this level of involvement, and some aren't able to participate actively. However, we might be surprised by the number of patients willing to engage with physicians in this way.

(2008, 35)

Given this, clinical decision-making entails distinguishable, yet interlocking, approaches that attempt to determine the presence of a clinical problem, its severity, and recommendations for treatment. While the clinician as a professional is charged with gathering and analyzing the data and recommending a plan of action according to accepted clinical methodologies, the patient plays a critical role in providing evidence and background for, and interpretation of, the clinical problem brought to the clinician's attention. There's no clinical problem and no decisions without a patient and clinician. Likewise, as we will explore, there's no clinical uncertainty without both parties.

Need for More Discussion on Clinical Uncertainty

As indicated above, there is a notable body of literature on clinical decision-making. It is based on how clinicians and patients make choices about what to attend to and how to respond in the clinical setting. Yet, the literature tends to focus on decision-making in the context of the search for *certainty*. Clinicians and patients search for certainty as they pursue evidence of signs and symptoms, causal relations, and probabilistic evidence in order to understand clinical problems and to determine reasonable treatments. Of course, they do. To suggest otherwise would undermine clinical knowledge and the methods used to arrive at "facts" about a clinical problem and recommendation for treatment. Pattern recognition brings together patient signs and symptoms for purposes of developing clinical descriptions and classifications that serve as treatment warrants. Causal or etiological analysis makes sense out of what brings a clinical problem about for purposes of treating or preventing it. Probabilistic analysis details quantitatively the extent to which a clinical problem is likely to occur within select patient populations. Nevertheless, none of these approaches grant certainty in medicine. Medical methodology cannot eliminate risk. Patterns of signs and symptoms can't always identify a specific clinical problem, etiological accounts are always oversimplified, and probabilistic analyses are always limited by the numbers. In each of the approaches reviewed above, there will be limits, ambiguity, disagreement, and trade-offs. It follows that seeking to know and do within a context of *clinical uncertainty* is far more the norm than the exception in medicine. Chapter 3 pursues this line as it explores the central role of uncertainty in clinical decision-making.

3 Clinical Uncertainty

Epistemological Roots

The Challenge of Clinical Uncertainty

When most of us think of clinical medicine, we think of a helping profession that delivers answers to our questions concerning our clinical problems. We think of a body of knowledge that describes and explains problems that individuals bring to the attention of health care professionals, forecasts what patients might experience, and serves as warrants for treatments and prevention. We think of a profession that has made possible the extension of the life span and enhanced quality of life during our lifetime. Yet, as we well know, clinical diagnosis, prognosis, treatment, and prevention are far from certain. As physician David M. Eddy says, "[u]ncertainty creeps into medical practice through every pore" (1984, 75). It creeps into the acts of "defining a disease, making a diagnosis, selecting a procedure, observing outcomes, assessing probabilities, assigning references, or putting it all together" (Eddy, 1984, 75). Defining a disease is not so easy because the line between normal and abnormal is often not clear (e.g., a moderate vs. severe case of COVID-19), some diseases are asymptomatic (e.g., asymptomatic vs. symptomatic COVID-19), and disease conditions (e.g., the flu and COVID-19) can share similar signs (e.g., a fever) and symptoms (e.g., fatigue) and yet differ in significant ways (e.g., the former caused by influenza viruses and the latter by SARS-CoV-2). Diagnoses can be less than certain because health care professionals do not and cannot know everything. Health care professionals can vary "in their ability to ask about symptoms, observe signs, interpret test results, and record the answers" (Eddy, 1984, 77). Selecting a procedure is no less difficult because there are typically "dozens of procedures that can be ordered" (Eddy, 1984, 78), and there is "variability in the people who perform procedures" (Eddy, 1984, 79). Observing outcomes is challenging because there are variations in how patients respond to medical interventions, clinicians typically do not follow patients over a long period of time, and some effects take years

DOI: 10.4324/9781032620978-3

to observe and evaluate (Eddy, 1984, 80–81). In the end, as Eddy says, clinical diagnosis and treatment recommendations

> must be done without knowing precisely what the patient has, with uncertainty about signs and symptoms, with imperfect knowledge of the sensitivity and specificity of tests, with no training in manipulating possibilities, with incomplete and biased information about outcomes, and with no language for communicating or assessing values.
>
> (1984, 83)

The bottom line is that uncertainty is not tangential to clinical decision-making; it is part and parcel of how and what we know in medicine (also see Fox, 1980; Mishel, 1988; Katz, 1984; Han, 2021).

The pandemic has brought us face-to-face with the reality of uncertainty in clinical decision-making. Recall the lengthy list of questions about our uncertainties about COVID-19 posed at the beginning of Chapter 1. Recall as well when Dr. Anthony Fauci, former member of the COVID-19 Task Force and Chief Medical Advisor to the President, was pressed by physician and Senator Rand Paul about being arrogant in his recommendations about masking, social distancing, and other matters during the pandemic. Note Fauci's response, one that is in keeping with the themes of this investigation of clinical uncertainty: "we don't know everything about this virus, and we really better be very careful" (Higgins-Dunn, 2020). Further, he said: "I am very careful and, hopefully, humble in knowing that I don't know everything about this disease and that's why I'm very reserved about making broad predictions" (Higgins-Dunn, 2020). Fauci goes on:

> I have never made myself out to be the end all and only voice in this. I'm a scientist, a physician, and a public health official. I give advice, according to the best scientific evidence. We should be humble about what we don't know.
>
> (Higgins-Dunn, 2020)

Let's heed the advice of Eddy and Fauci and consider the character of clinical uncertainty.

This chapter reviews some of the prominent literature on clinical uncertainty and distinguishes three dimensions of clinical uncertainty, namely, its source (or cause), issue (or problem), and locus (or stakeholder). Here, a source of uncertainty is probability, complexity, and ambiguity. An issue of uncertainty is lodged in scientific, practical, and personal contexts. A locus of uncertainty is a wide range of stakeholders (e.g., clinician, patient, family member, hospital administrator). The chapter illustrates intersections among the sources, issues, and loci of clinical uncertainty.

Such an account points in the direction of additional dimensions of clinical uncertainty that are developed in subsequent chapters.

The Notion of Uncertainty

The *Oxford English Dictionary* offers a number of definitions of uncertainty, two of which are relevant in this investigation. A first focuses on a state of mind of the knower. The *Oxford English Dictionary* says that uncertainty is "[t]he state or character of being *uncertain in mind*; a state of doubt; want of assurance or confidence; hesitation; irresolution" (1994, 2153, my italics). For instance, a clinician might say in 2021, "I am uncertain about how my patient will respond to the recommended COVID-19 treatment." Here the focus is on what is known by a knower, in this case, a clinician about COVID-19. *Oxford English Dictionary* also defines uncertainty in terms of the state of that which is known, namely, "*[s]omething* not definitely known or knowable" (1994, 2153, my italics). For instance, a patient might say in 2022, "The next variant of COVID-19 is uncertain." Here the focus is on the known, e.g., a variant of COVID-19. In both cases, one recognizes one's doubt about an object. To do this, one must be able to "step outside" oneself, so to speak, and reflect on what one knows. In this way, the cognitive state of uncertainty is a form "of 'metacognition'—a knowing about knowing" (Honigsbaum, 2019, 376). In this way, uncertainty is a state of conscious awareness of degree of doubt about something, some event, or person.

Taken together, uncertainty entails a state of the knower (e.g., a clinician) and a state of the known (e.g., a clinical problem). Let's take a moment to reflect on some assumptions here. In medicine, a state of uncertainty assumes a cognitive state of a clinician or patient who assumes that knowledge derives from quantifiable or qualifiable observations or experiences. An inability of a COVID-19 patient to breathe properly entails notable sensory experiences on the part of the patient. In this way, clinicians and patients are in part "philosophical empiricists" (see Wulff et al., 1986, 25ff). They each in their own way rely on sensory experience (e.g., touch, sight, sound, taste, smell) to arrive at knowledge claims about clinical problems. Correspondingly, a lack of such sensory experiences contributes to uncertainty in claims made about clinical problems. Not understanding why a former COVID-19 patient cannot breathe properly months after the infection has subsided indicates a lack of sensory experience and evidence about the clinical problem.

In addition, a state of uncertainty assumes the existence of an external world, in this case clinical problem such as disease, illness, deformity, or dysfunction. For the most part, clinicians and patients do not make up clinical problems. The disease, illness, deformity, or dysfunction associated with clinical problems are "real." An inability of a COVID-19 patient to breathe properly is not a figment of a clinician's and patient's imagination. It entails the experience of a tightening of the chest along with other symptoms. It entails degrees of dysfunction of the respiratory system. Given this, clinicians and patients are in part "philosophical realists" (see Wulff et al., 1986, 25ff). They each in their own way assume the existence of a clinical world outside them. Such a world is to be understood and perhaps manipulated given the evidence and technology that is available. Correspondingly, a lack of understanding and/or methods to change external agents that contribute to a clinical problem entails uncertainty in claims made about the clinical problem. Not understanding the particularities of lung dysfunction experienced by COVID-19 patients raises clinical uncertainties.

And, of course, this is oversimplified. Clinicians and patients are rarely either strict philosophical empiricists or philosophical realists. Clinical knowledge entails complex interactions between a knower and what is known. In the case of COVID-19, difficulty in breathing and evidence based on tests that a patient's lungs are not functioning properly go hand-in-hand in establishing clinical knowledge. Likewise, a lack of experience with a clinical problem and a lack of evidence about it creates uncertainty. Think of what little we knew about COVID-19 in 2016. While we knew about SARS, we had not yet experienced a different kind of SARS and had little evidence about SARS-CoV-2. The point is that clinical knowledge and clinical uncertainty emerge within the context of a complex interaction between a knower and a known.

Furthering the analysis, uncertainty entails degrees. Consider this continuum of degrees of knowledge (see Figure 3.1).

From the standpoint of the "I" as a knower, a "known known" is a state in which I know what is known. For instance, I know that SARS-CoV-2 is the virus that causes the disease COVID-19. In this state, my level of uncertainty is very low. An "unknown known" is a state in which I don't

known known	unknown known	known unknown	unknown unknown
"I know what's known."	"I don't know what's known"	"I know it's not known."	"I don't know it's not known."

Figure 3.1 Degrees of knowing.

know what is known. An example is that I know that I do not understand the genetics of SARS-CoV-2, while I would expect that Dr. Anthony Fauci does. In this state, my level of uncertainty is low insofar as I trust the knowledge source. A "known unknown" is a state in which I know something is not known. An example is that I know that there will be a pandemic in the future, but I and everyone else do not know what and when it will be. In this state, my level of uncertainty is higher. An "unknown unknown" is a state in which I don't know something is not known. An example is that I don't know what's not known about COVID-19. Insofar as I am aware of what I don't know, this is a category of uncertainty, and a high level at that. Insofar as I do not know what I do not know, this is not a category of uncertainty because I have no conscious awareness of doubt on a matter.

Of course, this is oversimplified. The relation between the known and the knower is mutually intertwined. We can know a lot about a clinical problem and at the same time be quite uncertain about its nature, etiology, prognosis, treatment, and prevention. In this way, knowledge of, and the corresponding uncertainties about, a clinical problem may defy being placed in any one of the categories. For instance, COVID-19 does not fit neatly into any one of the categories. It is neither a known known, an unknown known, a known unknown, nor an unknown unknown. It is rather some of each depending on what is known (e.g., about SARS-CoV-2), what is doubted (e.g., who will be affected), what emerges (e.g., about the post-acute sequelae of COVID-19), and what needs to be completely revised in light of new knowledge (e.g., long COVID is just a serious case of COVID-19). In this way, COVID-19 is characterized by what physician-philosopher Annemarie Mol (2002) calls in her work on philosophy of disease "multiple ontologies." Multiple ontologies refer to different expressions of a clinical problem. In her work, Mol focuses on atherosclerosis and explores how the clinical problem is framed diversely in patient information leaflets, imaging reports, doctor–patient conversations, and clinical case conferences. Such an ontological multiplicity does not, according to Mol, imply fragmentation. Instead, it implies coherence when one looks at it through the lens of clinical practice, the practice of caring for patients through informed clinical processes, and the assessment of the benefits and harms of alternative care options. In this way, multiple ontologies of a clinical problem entail multiple epistemologies, or ways of knowing. Such multiple ontologies and epistemologies serve to support coherent ways of knowing clinical problems, and they serve to support less-than-coherent ways and highlight the clinical uncertainties that are at stake.

In the case of COVID-19, COVID-19 is a heterogeneous clinical condition seen through the lens of virology, pulmonology, immunology, physiology, and genetics, among other specialties. Such ontological and epistemological multiplicities do not imply fragmentation, but rather different ways of framing a clinical problem for purposes of knowing and treating it. In these distinct, yet overlapping ways of knowing and doing, there will be coherence (e.g., in the case of explaining how a virus disrupts a patient's lung function) and there will be lots of questions (e.g., in the case of figuring out why some COVID-19 patients heal quickly and others struggle with the residual effects of the disease). Such multiple ontologies and epistemologies highlight how much we know about COVID-19 and the many ways we remain uncertain about this clinical condition. More is said about the intersectional character of clinical problems and our uncertainties in Chapter 5.

Clinical Uncertainty: Source, Issue, and Locus

Now that we have reflected a bit on uncertainty, how do we make sense out of different kinds of clinical uncertainty? Let's begin by taking a closer look at clinical uncertainty as it is discussed in the clinical literature. Physician Paul K.J. Han and his colleagues have devoted notable time to crafting taxonomies of clinical uncertainty (Han et al., 2011, 2017, 2019). They have distinguished a number of approaches to developing such taxonomies (Han et al., 2011). These include: (1) patient experiences of "uncertainty in illness" (Mishel, 1988) in terms of ambiguity of the illness, complexity of the treatments in the system of care, deficient information in the diagnosis, and unpredictability of the course of the illness and outcome; (2) expressions of uncertainty in health care (Babrow et al., 1998) in terms of the complexity of a clinical phenomenon, the quality of the clinical information, probability claims, the structure of clinical information, and lay understandings of clinical information; and (3) specific forms of uncertainty in particular fields in medicine (e.g., oncology) (Kasper et al., 2008) in terms of social integration, diagnosis and prognosis, deciphering information, mastering life changes, causal attribution, preferred degree of involvement in the patient–clinician interactions, clinicians' trustability, and efficacy of treatment.

   Building on the discussions, Han and his colleagues have developed an account of clinical uncertainty that reflects a number of its meanings: (a) a state of mind, (b) a state of being, (c) an object, and (d) a feature of an object (Han, 2021, 13). In the end, they find it sound to develop the epistemic character of clinical uncertainty in terms of its source, issue, and locus. As Han says,

   it is not the object or feature of the object that is uncertain; it is the human being who perceives and designates it as such. Uncertainty is ultimately a subjective rather than an objective phenomenon, a mental state rather than a material "thing" residing in the extra-mental world. It lies entirely in the eye and mind of the beholder.

(2021, 13–14)

We'll start with this interpretation and go from there.

Source

First, according to Han (2021), uncertainty arises from different *sources*. Here, a source

> consists of the origins of uncertainty, which can be conceived at two interconnected levels: (1) a proximate, superficial, informational level consisting of the symbolic representations of ignorance (the stimuli that engender uncertainty when encountered by individuals); and (2) an ultimate, deeper, conceptual level consisting of the root causes of ignorance (the actual sources of knowledge deficits that constitute the objects of uncertainty, but that normally remain latent and unacknowledged by individuals).
>
> (Han, 2021, 39)

At an informational level are three proximate sources of uncertainty: probability, complexity, and ambiguity. At a deeper, conceptual level are three corresponding ultimate root causes of ignorance: indeterminacy, intractability, and indeterminability (Han, 2021, 40). Let's consider each in turn.

Probability refers to risk, or "the existence or occurrence of some unknown current or future event" (Han, 2021, 40). It is a numerical estimate of how likely an event is to occur. An example of a probability statement is there is a "20% probability of benefit from treatment" (Han et al., 2011, 834). Such a statement is based on empirical or quantitative research of a population and estimates the number of individuals who express the outcome that is being studied. Earlier we considered an example of a probability statement heard in 2020 during the pandemic: "Although more than 80% of patients with COVID-19 infection have mild disease and make a full recovery, a significant proportion of patients progress to pneumonia, and half of these cases will develop severe acute respiratory syndrome (ARDS)" (Schleicher et al., 2020). This means that the probability that one will have mild symptoms is 80%, or eight out of ten. Twenty percent, or two out of ten, will have more severe symptoms.

At the root of probabilistic uncertainty is indeterminacy, "the lack of a definitive or fixed outcome or result" (Han, 2021, 41). Such is brought about by "the inherent *randomness* of natural processes, which makes future states fundamentally unknowable" (Han, 2021, 41, my italics). An example here is the inherent randomness in molecular processes of SARS-CoV-2 (Chen, 2020) as well as the host response of individuals to infection and therapeutic interventions (Han, 2021, 41). In addition, at the root of probabilistic uncertainty is "chaotic behavior" (Han, 2021, 41). Chaotic behavior comes about through nonlinear dynamics, feedback, and extreme sensitivity to initial conditions. Such are "defining features of 'complex adaptive systems'—collections of individual phenomenon that interact in multiple ways" (Han, 2021, 42). An example here is the chaotic behavior of COVID-19 during the course of the pandemic at the local, national, and global levels (Sapkota et al., 2021). As Sapkota et al. say,

> [t]he dynamics of the spread of pandemics are similar to the behavior of other nonlinear systems including chaotic maps and turbulent flows. In such systems, a small seed increases exponentially and then saturates; in general, chaotic behavior indicates that the system is extremely sensitive to the initial conditions.
>
> (2021, 80693)

Ambiguity is the quality of being open to more than one interpretation. Citing decision theorist Daniel Ellsberg (1961), Han defines ambiguity as a feature of risk information, "a quality depending on the amount, type, reliability, and 'unanimity,' of information, and giving rise to one's degree of 'confidence' in an estimate of relative likelihood" (Han, 2021, 42). In medicine, ambiguity is expressed quantitatively through risk ranges or confidence intervals around probabilities. Think here of the claim that SARS-CoV-2 testing entails 71%–98% sensitivity or the population-wide mortality rate from COVID-19 is .2%–1% (Han, 2021, 42–43). It can also be expressed qualitatively using terms such as "approximately" and "roughly" (Han, 2021, 43). In the case of COVID-19, ambiguity abounds, as found in the imprecision of data (e.g., for SARS-CoV-2 in Summer 2020), conflicting opinion about how to interpret evidence (e.g., the efficacy of boosters), and insufficient evidence (e.g., for "long COVID"). A debate that I have been following in my philosophy of death studies is whether a COVID-19 patient dies "of" or "with" COVID-19. Given that there is no accurate way to determine whether a death is primarily caused by COVID-19 or, let's say, a heart attack, the COVID-19 death rates can be said to be ambiguous (Hutto, 2022).

At the root of ambiguity is "indeterminability—the inability to establish a definitive or fixed outcome, result, or answer" (Han, 2021, 43). Indeterminacy arises from unreliability, incredibility, and inadequacy (Han, 2021, 43; also see Ellsberg, 1961). Unreliability "refers to shortcomings in the consistency and robustness of medical knowledge" (Han, 2021, 43).

An example here is the varying estimates of the accuracy and wide-effects of different COVID-19 vaccines. Incredibility "refers to shortcomings in the trustworthiness or believability of medical knowledge" (Han, 2021, 43). An example here is the contradictory guidance on social distancing put forth by various government officials and health experts. Inadequacy "refers to shortcomings in the amount of medical knowledge itself, which results from missing data or unmeasured variables" (Han, 2021, 43). An example here is the lack of existing information on long COVID or the lasting effects of SARS-CoV-2 infection on select populations of patients (e.g., the immune-compromised).

Complexity "refers to features of information that make it difficult to understand" (Han, 2021, 45). It "arises when informational elements increase in number, variety, or interconnectedness" (Han, 2021, 45). As an example, our knowledge of COVID-19 depends on multiple factors, such as nucleotide sequences and their related subfamilies (Chen, 2020), comorbidities, age, gender, class, race, ethnicity, and environmental factors (World Health Organization, 2020). COVID-19 provides an example of a disease condition in which an invading organism (i.e., the coronavirus called SARS-CoV-2), a host (i.e., the patient), and an environment (e.g., one that supports the survival of SARS-CoV-2) mutually contribute to the pathology of a disease condition. While SARS-CoV-2 causes COVID-19, there is more going on with regard to the expression of COVID-19. Sorting out the etiology, mechanisms, morphologies, and their functional consequences is critical in understanding COVID-19 and for developing therapeutic options.

At the root of complexity is "intractability—the resistance of a problem to human comprehension and control" (Han, 2021, 45). Intractability arises from two other sources. The first is "multiplicity in the components, attributes, or implications of a given problem" (Han, 2021, 45). An example is the multiple factors that lead to different expressions of COVID-19 (Rosén et al., 2022). The second is "interdependence between the components of a problem" (Han, 2021, 45–46). With COVID-19, multiple factors come together and contribute to its expressions. Sorting out the multiple factors and establishing their interdependence has yet to be worked out.

Issue

Second, according to Han (2021), uncertainty raises a number of *substantive issues*. Substantive issues are "specific, concrete problems, outcomes, situations, or alternatives that represent the objects of one's ignorance" (Han, 2021, 48). Han (2021, 48) isolates three main categories of substantive issues: scientific, practical, and personal. *Scientific uncertainty* "focuses on four main issues of medical problems: diagnosis, prognosis, cause, and treatment" (Han, 2021, 48). Think about debates about the diagnosis, prognosis, treatment, and prevention of COVID-19. We do not fully understand the SARS-CoV-2 variants, cannot predict with accuracy who will die from COVID-19, are unsure about how to treat long COVID, and do not have vaccines that fully prevent against COVID-19. While clinical professionals provide some answers to these questions, they cannot provide all answers because clinical methods, observations, and evidence are limited. They are limited because the information sources of clinical uncertainty, namely, probability, complexity, and ambiguity, and the conceptual sources, namely, indeterminacy, intractability, and indeterminability, are each limited.

Practical uncertainty pertains "to the structures and processes of healthcare" (Han, 2021, 50). One can be uncertain about the competence of a clinician, the reliability of clinical data, the quality of care, and how to navigate medical institutional issues. During the pandemic, we have heard concerns about the care of the elderly in assisted living, nursing homes, and long-term care facilities as care centers witnessed a disproportionate number of deaths from COVID-19 (National Consumer Voice for Quality Long-Term Care, 2021). We have questioned public health measures as we have balanced public health concerns with our need to work, spend time with family and friends, and visit our loved ones in hospitals and care facilities (Lowrey, 2021). We have encountered practical challenges regarding equitable and inclusive access to health care during the pandemic (Centers for Disease Control, 2021e). We have expressed mistrust of the medical profession during the pandemic when promises were broken; the distribution of resources was challenged; and we needed more from our health care providers, public health officials, and institutions (Bajaj and Stanford, 2021).

Personal uncertainty pertains "to psychosocial, economic, and existential concerns of both patients and clinicians" (Han, 2021, 51). One can be uncertain about the effects of one's disease or treatment on one's survival, lifestyle, and relationships. As previously mentioned, clinical data is based on population data and therefore clinicians and patients are left with determining how that population data applies to an individual case. These kinds of uncertainty can raise "existential" questions about the meaning and purpose of life as one reflects on how clinical data applies to oneself and how one ought to make clinical decisions in light of my own morbidity and mortality. During the COVID-19 pandemic, we witnessed stunning photos of patients dying alone in hospitals as well as dead bodies wrapped tightly in non-clear plastic wrap, transferred to refrigerator trucks, and buried in mass graves (Neilson, 2020). One worried that one would not see one's loved ones, and one would forego a funeral or memorial service if one died during the COVID-19 pandemic (Lowrey, 2021). Stress among health care workers was at an all-time high as they grappled with cases involving the distribution of scarce resources during a pandemic, policies regarding social distancing and isolation, and their own needs as members of families and communities. Many health care workers quit their jobs in late Spring and Summer 2021 during what has been called the "Great Resignation" in the U.S. (Gordon, 2022). The issues raised by our uncertainties during the pandemic were plentiful.

Locus

Third, uncertainty can have different *loci* (Han, 2021, 52). A locus refers "the person or persons in whose minds uncertainty—as the conscious metacognitive awareness of ignorance—resides" (Han, 2021, 52). Such persons or stakeholders include patients, their families and friends, health care providers, researchers, institutional administrators, regulators, payers, health policymakers, and the general public, among others. For instance, an individual who suspects she might have COVID-19 may be uncertain about whether to seek the attention of a health care professional for fear of getting sicker, receiving bad news, losing an income, or being asked to isolate from loved ones. A family member may be uncertain about whether to take a loved one to the doctor for fear of exposing the loved one to risky or uncertain care during the pandemic. A health care provider may be uncertain about the risks of going into work, entering a hospital room, and working with COVID-19 patients because of the risks of contagion for herself or loved ones and current or past ways in which the institution has not supported its workers. Stakeholders can have numerous and differing uncertainties depending on their perspectives, interests, and concerns.

Although it is helpful to distinguish loci of uncertainty, stakeholders typically work together. In the clinician–patient relationship, for instance, clinicians and patients can share uncertainty or "mutual ignorance" (Han, 2021, 53) with regard to a given medical problem. For instance, in February 2020, clinicians and patients mutually lacked knowledge about the new emerging clinical condition called COVID-19. Alternatively, clinicians and patients can be "equally aware (uncertain) of what they do not know about important issues of mutual concern" (Han, 2021, 54), a state called "shared uncertainty." For instance, in August 2022, clinicians and patients were mutually aware of uncertainties about the long-term effects of COVID-19. "Such symmetric, shared uncertainty is the ultimate goal of shared decision-making (SDM), an idealized process of care that promotes patient autonomy by facilitating the bidirectional transfer of information between clinicians and patients" (Han, 2021, 54). In between "mutual ignorance" and "shared uncertainty" are situations of "unilateral uncertainty," where "one party resides in a state of ignorance, [and] the other in a state of uncertainty—that is, consciously aware of his or her ignorance" (Han, 2021, 53). One thinks here of a situation in which a clinician is aware of uncertainty about the effectiveness of monoclonal antibody therapy for early COVID-19 and the patient is not able to process such information, or a patient is aware of uncertainty about following recommended treatment protocols because of their own situational constraints and the clinician is not aware of such constraints. There were plenty of loci of uncertainty during the pandemic.

Intersections Among Source, Issue, and Locus

According to Han, the source, issue, and locus of uncertainty interrelate (2021, 55). An uncertainty about a substantive issue (e.g., a scientific, practical, or personal one) can be framed by uncertainty about informational sources (e.g., probability, ambiguity, or complexity). Different stakeholders (e.g., clinicians, patients, family members, hospital administration) can be uncertain about different substantive issues or informational sources (e.g., a diagnosis, response to treatment, impact on family life, impact on the budget). As an example, a 65-year-old COVID-19 patient can experience uncertainty about her ability to breathe, her response to treatment, her change of recovery and survival, the competence of her clinicians, the impact of illness on her family, and her financial well-being after missing many days from work. Simultaneously, a clinician can experience uncertainty about the diagnosis, prognosis, and treatment options for her 65-year-old COVID-19 patient as new knowledge about probabilities and complexity of COVID-19 emerge in the clinical literature and are shared among colleagues. Simultaneously, hospital administrators can experience uncertainty about the pandemic's toll on staffing, resource allocation, and finances on the institution. The point is that the epistemic dimensions of clinical uncertainty intersect in various ways. This is an important point that will be developed at greater length in subsequent chapters.

Probability, Ambiguity, and Complexity

As featured above, Han gives us insight into the epistemic or knowledge-based roots of clinical uncertainty that are evident in our discussion of COVID-19. Here are three considerations about the epistemology of clinical uncertainty that we will continue to develop:

1 We are uncertain because clinical knowledge is probabilistic. It entails an indeterminacy of a definitive or fixed outcome or result.

2 We are uncertain because clinical knowledge is ambiguous. It is unreliable, non-credible, or inadequate.
3 We are uncertain because clinical knowledge is complex. It is multidimensional and interdependent.

These lessons will serve as focal points in the upcoming analysis as we continue to unpack the epistemological character of clinical uncertainty. Han's lessons on the substantive and loci-based issues come into play in the context of a wider frame of understanding of clinical uncertainty offered in subsequent chapters. As will be shown, forecasting future discussions, substantive issues, and loci entail more than epistemic considerations; they entail ontological and evaluative ones.

Need for a Wider Lens of Clinical Uncertainty

As one can see, clinical knowledge is epistemically uncertain. It is epistemically uncertain in that knowledge is probabilistic, ambiguous, and complex. It is also uncertain because it is framed by claims and assumptions about clinical problems and the evaluations made of them by professionals who seek to treat them. Chapter 4 explores further levels, kinds, and dimensions of clinical uncertainty in order to provide a broader sense of its notion.

4 Clinical Uncertainty

Ontological and Axiological Roots

There's More to the Story

So far, our investigation leads us to appreciate the uncertainty of knowledge in clinical medicine. On this view, clinical knowledge is limited by the constraints of the knower, the methods by which knowledge is acquired, and the data itself. But there's more to the story. Clinical knowledge offers an ontology of clinical nature, i.e., an account of the nature of clinical problems in light of its limits, changes, and complexities. Further, clinical knowledge is prescriptive; it guides actions in medicine. Such actions are framed by values, which are ambiguous, varied, and chosen. This chapter investigates clinical uncertainty through discussions in the philosophy of medicine and shows how clinical uncertainty is not simply an epistemological phenomenon, it is an ontological and axiological one. Here "philosophy of medicine" is a branch of philosophy that explores issues in theory, research, and practice within the fields of the health sciences (Broadbent, 2019; Stegenga, 2018; Thompson and Upshur, 2017; Gøtzsche and Wulff, 2007; Marcum, 2008; Pellegrino, 2008; Engelhardt, 1996; Reznek, 1987; Wulff et al., 1986). Philosophy of medicine is by its design interdisciplinary and draws from literature in clinical medicine, psychology, communication, history, sociology, anthropology, and political science in mapping out the terrain of ideas, concepts, and values in medicine. The literature that follows points to important areas of reflection on clinical uncertainty that often are absent in the clinical literature.

Clinical Uncertainty: Nature and Values

The Uncertainty of Clinical Problems: Limit, Change, Complexity

As we saw in Chapter 3, knowledge of disease entails epistemic commitments in terms of the sources of knowledge, the issues that are raised, and the stakeholders that make knowledge claims. In medicine,

DOI: 10.4324/9781032620978-4

we know through empirical or sense-based frames of reference that are organized theoretically, through theories and methods of inference that bring order to the theories. In the case of COVID-19, we know COVID-19 through observations and tests, and the theoretical frames that make sense out of the virus we call SARS-CoV-2 and its spread in human populations. The epistemological claims we make about clinical problems and COVID-19 work hand-in-hand with ontological commitments regarding claims and assumptions about clinical problems as phenomena of the natural world. Here, "ontological" (or as some might say, "metaphysical") concerns the nature of things, of what exists. Clinical knowledge attempts to make sense of clinical nature and, in so doing, it advances views about it. In this way, there is a widespread assumption in medicine that clinical nature exists in part independently of the clinical knower, and such reality stimulates our senses to arrive at accounts of clinical problem. In other words, clinicians and patients don't make clinical problems up. Of course, they don't. Think of the pain and suffering or loss of function and well-being that we experience when ill that is neither a choice nor a figment of one's imagination. When I had COVID-19 for the first time in February 2023 and could not breathe easily, I certainly did not choose this experience, especially during a record ski year in Colorado. The difficulty I experienced breathing was not a figment of my imagination as I struggled to climb a snow-covered mountain during my usual mid-day walk at 8,000 feet of elevation. While we may agree that the clinical classifications and descriptions of clinical problems are in part created by our perceptions and languages, we do not make them up. Lung dysfunction, viral infection, and fever are "real." In this way, clinical knowers are typically "philosophical realists," who hold that there is an external world, or clinical nature, that is based on phenomena outside of our perception and control (Wulff et al., 1986). It follows that discussion of the ontology of a clinical problem is relevant in a discussion of clinical uncertainty.

As clinical professionals and patients can be uncertain of the claims they make about clinical problems, they can also be uncertain about the objects, structures, and mechanisms that they encounter in clinical practice. Physicians Christof Tannert and his colleagues say that

> ontological uncertainty is caused by the *stochastic features of a situation*, which will usually involve complex technical, biological, and/or social systems. Such complex systems are often characterized by non-linear behaviour, which makes it impossible to resolve uncertainties by deterministic reasoning and/or research.
>
> (2007, 893, my italics)

Similarly, Han agrees with system scientists Rueben McDaniel and Dean Driebe (2001) that "*chaotic behavior is part of the natural order of the universe,* and cannot be avoided, eliminated, or controlled. In other words, indeterminacy is ultimately ontological in nature—rooted in the *basic structures of reality*—and fundamentally irreducible" (2021, 42, my italics).

Clinical problems are not simply complex; they defy being known fully, thus contributing to clinical uncertainty. French philosopher Michel Foucault (1973 [1963]) illustrates four distinguishable attributes of disease: (1) complexity of combination, (2) analogy, (3) frequency, and (4) calculation of degrees of certainty. First, what we call a disease expresses a complex configuration of experience that is "related, more or less directly, to essences whose increasing generality guaranteed a decreasing complexity: the class was simpler than the species, which, in turn, was simpler than the actual, immediate disease" (Foucault, 1973 [1963], 99). For instance, the disease we call COVID-19 is based on shared perceptions of cases of signs, symptoms, and test results (e.g., fever, body aches, and respiratory distress) as reported by patients in the clinic. Given this, what we call a disease will always be "simpler" than individual expressions of that which is described, classified, diagnosed, predicted, treated, and prevented. As a consequence, there will be variations in disease expression because disease categories and descriptions are not a "one size fits all" of that which presents in the clinic. Think of the different signs and symptoms and responses to treatments, vaccines, and boosters that COVID-19 patients have reported during their illnesses. Some had multiple symptoms and others had none. Some had persistent coughs and others had headaches. Others responded well to Paxlovid and others did not. Some never got COVID-19 after vaccination and others did. This reminds us that the disease we call COVID-19 is not one thing; it is a heterogenous clinical condition. A disease category brings together the complexity of combinations of shared clinical phenomena.

Second, what we call disease expresses analogies.

> The analogies on which the clinical gaze [i.e., the clinical perception] rested in order to recognize, in different patients, signs and symptoms, are of a different order; they "consist in the relations that exist first between the constitutive [i.e., contributing] parts of a single disease, and between a known disease and a disease to be known."
>
> (Foucault, 1973 [1963], 100)

In other words, what we call disease entails analogies or comparisons between what we know about a newly emerging disease in the light of similar ones, seen through the frame of a "clinical gaze." Here, the clinical gaze refers to how clinicians perceive what is reported by patients and then fit their perceptions into interpretations of the disease, in the context of a biomedical paradigm, with its assumptions about space (e.g., size, composition) and time (e.g., causality, degree). For instance, analogies between COVID-19 and previously discovered clinical problems (e.g., SARS) are made in order to draw from what we have learned about coronaviruses as well as to distinguish a "novel" clinical event from previous ones. Further, analogies between clinical conditions are made in order to assist in forecasting future clinical conditions, ones that are known to us as well as those that we have yet to know, such as the coronaviruses that will bring about the next pandemic.

Third, what we call disease expresses a perception of frequencies, or rate at which something occurs. As Foucault says, "[m]edical knowledge will gain in certainty only in relation to the number of cases examined" (1973 [1963], 101). Such is a message familiar to any student in science or medicine today: sample size matters. On this view, disease is an accumulation of evidence, which changes as new evidence arises and is integrated into existing ways of knowing. The clinical gaze fits the patient's story into a biomedical paradigm and prioritizes biomedical information, an approach that has proven to be quite effective as evidenced by the success of evidence-based medicine. For instance, COVID-19 is based on the frequency of the cases that are observed and treated, which are submitted to investigation and discussion and serve as a basis for our clinical descriptions, classifications, and explanations.

Fourth, what we call disease entails a calculation of degrees of certainty. Citing physician Charles-Louis Dumas (1765–1803), Foucault says,

> [i]f one day one discovered in the calculation of probability a method that might be suitably adapted to complicated objects, to abstract ideas, to variable elements in medicine and physiology, one would soon produce the highest degree of certainty, to which the sciences can attain.
> (1973 [1963], 103)

And even then, one is never certain. "Total *description* [of a disease] is a present and ever-withdrawing horizon; it is much more the dream of thought than a basic conceptual structure" of reality (Foucault, 1973 [1963], 115, my italics). It is much more the dream because "[m]edical certainty must be obtained by a combination of probabilities" (Foucault, 1973 [1963], 116). Because such combinations are never fully obtained, we are left with uncertainty in medicine. On this view, COVID-19 represents degrees of certainty (or uncertainty) in the calculations that are made about probabilities, analogies, and frequencies of a clinical problem. That's it. Such calculations are the best we can do, but they are also quite useful in that they lead to evidence-based medicine as opposed to pseudo-clinical practice. Further, they require that we imagine, question, and enter into reflection and dialogue in clinical medicine (Engebretsen, 2016, 601).

Given that what we call disease turns on the complexity of combination, analogy, frequency, and calculation of degrees of certainty, Foucault says the following:

> we must abandon the idea of an ideal, transcendent Spectator whose genius and patience might be approached to a greater or lesser degree by real observers. *The only normative observer is the totality of observers*: the errors produced by their individual points of view are distributed in a totality that possesses its own powers of indication.
>
> (1973 [1963], 102, my italics)

In other words, in medicine, what we call disease represents the observations and reportings of a totality of clinical observers, set within the context of a biomedical paradigm and accepted professional clinical standards of the time. For instance, the disease we call COVID-19 reflects the observations and reportings of clinicians and patients, interpreted within the context of twenty-first-century infectious disease paradigms and accepted clinical standards.

Indeed, Foucault draws our attention to important epistemological roots of clinical uncertainty. He reminds us that "the only normative observer [in medicine] is the totality of observers (Foucault, 1973 [1963], 102). In other words, the standard or norm for knowledge in contemporary medicine is not the all-knowing person, but rather the totality of clinical observers. Yet, I think, Foucault goes further, drawing our attention to the ontological roots of disease. Disease is constituted by clinical observations of signs and symptoms, analogies between similar clinical expressions, frequencies of rates of clinical events, and calculations of degrees of accuracy. In this way, disease is illusive (in terms of an account of knowledge in which all-knowing is possible), changing, and complex. In the case of COVID-19, we'll never fully understand "it," for "it" evolves and entails multiple factors and expressions in nature. But there is still an "it" that lends itself to clinical classification and description, treatment, research, and funding. We do not simply make it up in the clinical world. Pain and suffering are "real." Clinical treatment "really" works. And clinical nature will have its way, regardless sometimes of how we understand it and what we do to change it.

Given this, Foucault gives us three considerations about the ontological character of clinical uncertainty that we will continue to develop in this investigation:

1 We are uncertain because a clinical problem cannot fully be known. A clinical problem is limited by our clinical frames of reference.
2 We are uncertain because a clinical problem changes. It changes in terms of space (e.g., size, composition) and time (e.g., causality, degree).
3 We are uncertain because a clinical problem is complex. It is multidimensional and interdependent.

These lessons will serve as focal points in the upcoming analysis as we unpack the ontological character of clinical uncertainty.

The Uncertainty of Clinical Values: Ambiguity, Variation, and Choice

In that there is no "transcendent" clinical knower and clinical object in nature, the uncertainties that arise provide a multitude of opportunities in medicine. They guide what we *ought* to do in medicine. As we saw in the previous chapter and section, knowledge of disease entails ontological commitments regarding the structure of clinical nature. In the case of COVID-19, the epistemological claims we make about clinical problems and COVID-19 work hand-in-hand with ontological commitments regarding claims and assumptions about its clinical nature. Correspondingly, knowledge and nature uncertainty occur when one is doubtful about one's knowledge about something or some event, e.g., whether a COVID-19 patient would benefit clinically from being put on a ventilator. Here the focus is on uncertainty about verifiable facts (Sepielli, 2009). Further, the epistemological and ontological claims work hand-in-hand with axiological commitments, regarding what ought to be done in medicine. In the case of COVID-19, understanding a viral condition that has led to 43% more deaths in June 2020 serves to guide treatment and prevention (Hutto, 2022). The development of therapeutic and preventive measures is guided by evidence-based considerations as well as the goals to minimize pain and suffering and to promote health and well-being. Such goals are evaluative and focused on what is good and right in the lives of patients. Correspondingly, value uncertainty concerns uncertainty about the *reasons* verifiable facts give us (Sepielli, 2009). In the case of COVID-19, value uncertainty can occur when one asks whether putting one patient on a ventilator as opposed to another patient is reasonable in terms of what is the "right" action to take or what one ought to do. In this way, epistemological and ontological claims about clinical nature are framed by axiological or evaluative considerations.

Physician and biomedical ethicist H. Tristram Engelhardt, Jr. (1941–2018) (1996) helps us understand the axiological sense of clinical knowledge and nature. Here, axiology is the study of values and includes questions concerning the nature and classification of values or claims of worth. Engelhardt has long defended the view that clinical knowledge is value-ladened. As he says,

> [o]ne will not be able simply to discover, by appeal to factual issues alone, what treatments are indicated, what treatments are appropriate, what treatments are ordinary, or what treatments are extraordinary. Integral to such judgments will be appeals to particular hierarchies of values and to peaceable processes for resolving disputes in these matters.
>
> (Engelhardt, 1996, 221)

In the case of COVID-19, for instance, one will not be able simply to discover by appeal to factual issues alone, which diagnoses, prognoses, treatments, and preventions are indicated and which ones are not. One will need to consider available evidence, current thinking and guidelines in the profession, the goals that are sought to be achieved, and the ethical implications of one's actions.

Determining a diagnosis, prognosis, treatment, and prevention involves appeals to what goals or consequences *ought* to be achieved in medicine. As Engelhardt puts it, "[p]roblems stand as problems for medicine because they are disvalued" (1996, 203). For instance, the condition we call COVID-19 harms us, and thus we seek to minimize, if not eradicate, the effects the virus has on our health and in our lives. Further, "[t] he very appreciation of a problem as a problem for medicine is tied to its appearing as a failure to achieve a desired state" (Engelhardt, 1996, 203). For instance, humans typically desire to socialize with others, and COVID-19 compromises the ability to be physically close to our loved ones. The very appreciation of a problem as a problem for medicine "may be a failure to achieve a desired or expected level of freedom from pain or anxiety" (Engelhardt, 1996, 203). For instance, COVID-19 often entails pain in the chest and anxiety with regard to how one will be affected by this. The very appreciation of a problem as a problem for medicine "may involve a failure to achieve an expected level of function" (Engelhardt, 1996, 203). For instance, COVID-19 typically entails a problem in the "normal" functioning of the lungs. The very appreciation of a problem as a problem for medicine "may involve a failure to achieve an expected realization of human form or grace" (Engelhardt, 1996, 203). Consider that a failure to breathe properly is not in keeping with desired human form. Not allowing loved ones to visit their hospitalized relatives, burying COVID-19 patients in mass graves, and prohibiting end-of-life services are not in keeping with human grace in secular and spiritual traditions. The very appreciation of a problem as a problem for medicine "may involve a failure to achieve what is an expected span of life" (Engelhardt, 1996,

203). Early and sudden death from COVID-19 is typically not desired. Taken together, "[t]hese genres of judgments [in medicine] depend on a family of values; they characterize circumstances as ones of suffering, of pathology, or as a problem to be solved" (Engelhardt, 1996, 204).

In addition to consequential or goal-oriented evaluations of goals, there is another major set of values that frame our decisions in clinical decision-making. These arise from human choice, the act of selecting or making a decision when faced with one or more options. In democratic cultures, patients and health care practitioners have choices. Patients choose whether to make appointments with health care professionals and health care professionals choose to treat patients. Patients choose among a host of options involving treatment and health care professionals choose among options for screens, tests, and recommendations. The ability to choose is a basis for the ethical principles of autonomy, patient rights, and employee rights. It is a basis for a "morality of mutual respect grounded in permission" (Engelhardt, 1996, 122) and the moral practice of informed consent in the clinical setting. In this practice, choice-makers ought to be respected in the moral community, and choice-makers are owed certain kinds of treatment, such as the provision of information, protection of bodily and mental integrity, and avenues for making claims when violations occur.

In addition, choice-makers ought to be able to decline information. As Engelhardt says, "[p]articular patients, if they decline such knowledge, need not be told what rational and prudent individuals (within a particular community with its particular moral vision) usually need to know in order to make a reasonable decision" (1996, 316). As he says,

> [b]oth *Cobbs v. Grant* and *Sardy v. Hardy*, for example, explicitly underscore that a physician is not obligated to disclose risks when the patient requests not to be informed. The right to be informed is not an obligation to be informed. Nor does it create an overriding obligation on the part of the physician to inform. It rather requires offering to the patient the opportunity to acquire information.
>
> (Engelhardt, 1996, 316)

In the case of COVID-19, any patient would be able to decline clinical information, tests, and treatments, all within the boundaries of local, regional, state, and federal law governing practices during the pandemic. In addition, any patient may decline clinical information, sign consent documents, and ask the clinician to proceed as she would for any patient in a similar situation.

An implication here is that clinical decision-makers ought to be able to choose to be uncertain. We can all relate to someone who, in 2020, said she did not want to know whether she had COVID-19 because there was little that could be done. We can all relate to someone who, in 2021, said she was uncertain about venturing into a health care facility for tests in order to avoid contracting COVID-19. We can all relate to someone who, in 2022, said that she was uncertain about being boostered because she previously contracted COVID-19 and believes that her prior infection brought about sufficient immunization. We can all relate to someone who, in 2023, contracted COVID-19 after being vaccinated and boostered and then reported that she is uncertain about whether the vaccine and boosters worked. Putting aside those who have a moral (and legal) duty to know (e.g., a clinician who cares for a patient), clinical decision-makers as moral agents can ethically choose not to know, and thereby remain uncertain about their health status.

Given this, there will be variations among clinical decision-makers with regard to comfort with uncertainty. According to Engelhardt, "[t]his underscores the circumstance that different individuals seek different sorts of physician-patient relationships. Some wish to be full collaborators in their treatment, if not directly control it" (1996, 316). I suspect that many of my readers find themselves in this camp and seek to be informed about their clinical conditions and the options before them.

> On the other hand, many wish to entrust their care to a physician in which they have faith. Such individuals wish last and least of all to be obliged to listen to all the risks and possible harms to which they may be subjected.
>
> (Engelhardt, 1996, 316)

I suspect that we all know of someone who chose this option.

And then there are situations in which others choose for us, a phenomenon that I call "manufactured uncertainty." These situations can range from outright violation of respect for the choice-maker to "caring" paternalistic intervention. One thinks here of the case of a government that restricts its citizens from researching COVID-19 in order to control messages during the pandemic (Lei and Qiu, 2020). On a smaller scale, one thinks of a case involving withholding clinical information from a competent patient because the patient is experiencing information overload or emotional turmoil. As Engelhardt tells us,

> [o]ne will need in medicine, as in everyday life, to distinguish between acts of coercion and those of peaceful manipulation. If one understands coercive actions as those that place or threaten to place a patient in a disadvantaged state without justification, and if one defines peaceable manipulation as those actions that place or offer to place a patient in an

advantaged state to which the patient is not entitled, coercions will be forbidden and peaceable manipulations will be allowed.

(1996, 308)

The first violates the morality of mutual respect by violating the free choice of innocent persons, but the second does not. More is said about such ethical issues in Chapter 7.

The challenge with evaluative judgments in medicine is that they are often uncertain in ways that go beyond choosing to be uncertain. Evaluative judgments are uncertain because they can be ambiguous (e.g., unclear or lack reasons); can vary in terms of kind (e.g., goals and choices), direction (positive or negative), or degree (strong or weak); and can be at odds with other choice-makers (and thereby bring about moral conflict or moral distress). In the case of COVID-19, one may be accepting of significant limits on one's freedom in order to protect one's loved ones and members of the public. Another may be accepting of contracting COVID-19 in order to see one's loved ones in the hospital or nursing home. One may invoke a right to choose not to vaccinate based on religious exemptions (e.g., National Catholic Bioethics Center, 2021), while another may support mandatory vaccination for all workers on the basis of public health concerns (Thagard, 2021). One can be positive or negative in one's value commitment, and one can have strong or weak reactions in one's evaluation, such as we witnessed in discussions about mandatory masking during the pandemic. Evaluative judgments vary in ways that reflect a rich array of value judgments.

Yet, all is not relative. As Engelhardt says, "[t]here are circumstances likely to be disvalued in whatever culture an individual lives, and in terms of whatever goals are possessed by individuals or societies" (1996, 204). There will be circumstances that will likely be disvalued in nearly any foreseeable environment (e.g., caring for loved ones) and in terms of any likely cluster of human purposes (e.g., living without pain and suffering). In the case of COVID-19, many have expressed concerns about social isolation during COVID-19 and especially in the context of dying alone without loved ones by the side (Lowrey, 2021; Nelson-Becker and Victor, 2020). For another example, many have said that we could have done a better job during the pandemic distributing medical resources (e.g., PPEs, beds, vaccines) to those in need (Foxwell, 2022). While moral agents express a variety of value commitments, they also find points of agreement on the goals and duties that are morally binding.

Nevertheless, the challenges that arise in managing clinical uncertainty are rooted in the uncertain nature of clinical values. As much as we may seek certainty in our values, certainty is not forthcoming. Values are ambiguous, can vary, and are a function of our choices, which change and evolve. In clinical medicine, it is no different. Clinical values are ambiguous (e.g., to treat or not to treat a futile patient), can vary (e.g., respect patient autonomy vs. advance the patient's best interest), and are chosen (e.g., my choice vs. your choice). In this way, Engelhardt gives us insight into the axiological roots of clinical uncertainty that are applicable to our discussion of COVID-19. Here, there are three considerations that we will build on:

1 We are uncertain because clinical values are ambiguous. They are unclear or lack reasons.
2 We are uncertain because clinical values vary. They vary in kind (e.g., goal vs. choice), direction (e.g., positive or negative), or degree (e.g., strong or weak).
3 We are uncertain because we choose to be uncertain or others choose that we are uncertain.

These lessons will serve as focal points in the upcoming analysis as we continue to unpack the axiological character of clinical uncertainty.

Need for an Expanded Taxonomy of Clinical Uncertainty

The account of clinical uncertainty that results from literature in the philosophy of medicine recognizes that clinical knowledge is framed by clinical nature and the evaluations we make of it. Correspondingly, epistemic uncertainty is framed by ontological and axiological uncertainty. Chapter 5 brings together levels, kinds, and dimensions of clinical uncertainty that are developed in this and the prior chapter in order to offer an expanded and intersectional taxonomy of clinical uncertainty.

5 A Taxonomy of Clinical Uncertainty

An Expanded and Integrative Account of Clinical Uncertainty

This investigation of clinical uncertainty is not simply an academic or conceptual one; it is a practical one. As Hans et al. say, "From a clinical standpoint, the principle value of the new taxonomy is as a means of facilitating the diagnosis and management of the uncertainties that arise in clinical practice" (2011, 835). I am in agreement with Han et al. that a taxonomy of clinical uncertainty has immense practical import. An account of clinical uncertainty can provide practical guidelines to clinicians and patients about what to look for in considering clinical evidence, a clinical problem, and treatment options in the context of shared and differing clinical values. Yet, parting with Han et al. (2011), I would like to see a broader taxonomy of clinical uncertainty than what is offered in the clinical literature and one that accounts for the wider range of clinical uncertainties that clinicians and patients encounter. I would also like to see an intersectional account of clinical uncertainty, one that recognizes the forces that frame clinical decision-making.

Given discussions in Chapters 3 and 4, this chapter calls for an expanded and intersectional account of clinical uncertainty. It calls for an appreciation of clinical uncertainty that goes beyond the epistemological focus that is predominant in the clinical literature to include ontological and axiological considerations. The chapter offers an expanded taxonomy of clinical uncertainty in terms of philosophical levels (i.e., epistemological, ontological, and axiological), kinds of clinical uncertainty (i.e., clinical knowledge, clinical nature, and clinical value), and dimensions of uncertainty (i.e., probabilistic, evidence ambiguity, evidence complexity, transcendent, nature-change, nature complexity, value-ambiguity, value-kind, and choice). Further, it illustrates how levels, kinds, and dimensions of uncertainty intersect in clinical decision-making within situated frames of contexts and identities (e.g., age, sex/gender, race/ethnicity, caregiver role/

DOI: 10.4324/9781032620978-5

the care for role, class/economic status, social role/empowerment, ability/disability, religion/spirituality).

A Taxonomy of Clinical Uncertainty

The prior two chapters consider a number of ways to understand uncertainty in clinical decision-making. In Chapter 3, Han (2021) reminds us that uncertainty in clinical medicine arises in three ways, namely, through its source, issue, and locus. He draws our attention to epistemological considerations and illustrates how clinical knowledge is uncertain because it is probabilistic, ambiguous, and complex. In Chapter 4, Foucault (1973 [1963]) reminds us that uncertainty in medicine arises from an ontology of clinical problems. Clinical problems themselves are complex and seen through what Foucault calls the "clinical gaze." While the clinical gaze emphasized the role of perception in how we know, it gazes *toward* something or some event, such as a clinical problem. Of interest here is that clinical uncertainty arises from the illusive, changing, and complex nature of clinical problems. In Chapter 4 as well, Engelhardt (1996, Ch. 5) reminds us that uncertainty in medicine arises from the role values play in clinical knowledge and action. He draws our attention to axiological considerations and how clinical knowledge and the problems that we know are understood through evaluative frameworks. Clinical uncertainty arises because values are ambiguous, can vary in kind, and are chosen.

Given this, we arrive at an expanded taxonomy of clinical uncertainty in decision-making. While there can be more and different classifications in the taxonomy, we'll focus in this investigation on three philosophical levels, three kinds, and nine dimensions to draw our attention to a wider lens on clinical uncertainty, one that entails epistemic, ontological, and evaluative considerations. Again, that's the point: a taxonomy of clinical uncertainty will need to address assumptions and claims about clinical problems as well as the role values play in their constructions and applications in practice. Putting this together, we arrive at the following taxonomy of clinical uncertainty, along with examples drawn from the COVID-19 pandemic (see Table 5.1).

In this world of clinical uncertainty, so to speak, we do not know everything about a clinical problem, we cannot know everything about it, and there can be value disagreement about what ought to be done about the clinical problem, especially when the stakes are high. Consider the following case of COVID-19 from a New Jersey hospital published in May 2020 prior to an approved treatment plan for COVID-19 (Douedi and Miskoff, 2020). The case involves a 77-year-old female with a history of hypertension and hyperlipidemia who presented as a transfer to a hospital with worsening fever, cough, and respiratory distress. As reported, "chest

Table 5.1 A taxonomy of clinical uncertainty

Philosophical level	Kind	Dimension	Example of statement	Example from the COVID-19 pandemic
Epistemological uncertainty	Clinical knowledge uncertainty	Probabilistic uncertainty	We are uncertain because clinical knowledge is probabilistic.	"I am uncertain because I do not know if I will be in the 20% of those hospitalized for COVID-19 if I become infected."
		Evidence-ambiguity uncertainty	We are uncertain because clinical knowledge is ambiguous.	"I am uncertain about which prevention recommendations to follow because they appear at odds."
		Evidence-complexity uncertainty	We are uncertain because clinical knowledge is complex.	"I am uncertain about how risk factors (e.g., co-morbidities) play a role in the severity of my COVID-19 illness."
Ontological uncertainty	Clinical problem uncertainty	Transcendent uncertainty	We are uncertain because a clinical problem cannot fully be known.	"COVID-19 is not one disease, and thus I am uncertain about what I have."
		Nature-change uncertainty	We are uncertain because a clinical problem changes.	"COVID-19 changes with each variant, and thus I am uncertain about what I have."
		Nature-complexity uncertainty	We are uncertain because a clinical problem is complex.	"COVID-19 is complex, and thus I am uncertain about what I have."

(Continued)

Table 5.1 (Continued)

Philosophical level	Kind	Dimension	Example of statement	Example from the COVID-19 pandemic
Axiological uncertainty	Clinical value uncertainty	Value–ambiguity uncertainty	We are uncertain because clinical values are ambiguous.	"I am uncertain about consenting to a new COVID-19 intervention without knowing more about the clinical side-effects or harms."
		Value-kind uncertainty	We are uncertain because clinical values vary.	"I am uncertain about what to do because my duty to prevent the spread of COVID-19 conflicts with my duty to bring in an income to provide for my family."
		Choice uncertainty	We are uncertain because we choose to be uncertain or others choose that we are uncertain.	"I am uncertain because I don't want to know whether I have COVID-19 because there is no effective way to treat it." "I am uncertain because I do not know if authorities are telling us what they know or don't know."

X-rays revealed bilateral infiltrates worse at the lung bases and CT scan of the chest showed bilateral ground-glass opacities consistent with COVID-19" (Douedi and Miskoff, 2020). Testing in a previous facility revealed a positive result, while testing at the current facility revealed a negative one. The patient

> was treated aggressively in the intensive care unit with high dose intra-venous ascorbic acid, hydroxychloroquine, and anti-interleukin-6 monoclonal antibody. She also received a loading dose of remdesivir [,] however was unable to complete the course due to organ failure and requirement of vasopressors for hemodynamic stability.
>
> (Douedi and Miskoff, 2020)

Following this, the patient remained critically ill and was eventually placed on comfort care per the family's wishes, and passed away soon after. Clinicians report the following "lessons":

> With a rapidly growing death rate and more than 200,000 confirmed cases worldwide, COVID-19 has become a global pandemic and major hit to our healthcare systems. While several companies have already begun vaccine trials and healthcare facilities have been using a wide-range of medications to treat the virus and symptoms, there is not yet an approved medication regime for COVID-19 infections. The alarming increase in cases per day adds an additional pressure to find a cure and decrease the global health burden and mortality rate.
>
> (Douedi and Miskoff, 2020)

This case illustrates a number of dimensions of clinical uncertainty:

1 *probabilistic uncertainty*: The case occurs in May 2020 and in the early stages of the pandemic. Probability estimates about recommended treatments and survival rates are limited in the clinical literature adding to the challenge of interpreting probabilistic data for a clinical problem.
2 *evidence-ambiguity uncertainty*: During the time of the case, there is debate, disagreement, and limited evidence on "an approved medica-tion regime" (Douedi and Miskoff, 2020). This leads to uncertainty and a call "to find a cure and decrease the global health burden and mortality rate" (Douedi and Miskoff, 2020).
3 *evidence-complexity uncertainty*: In May 2020, there is anecdotal evi-dence that the elderly are more vulnerable to COVID-19, but limited evidence about what and how comorbidities play a role in COVID-19 expression in elderly populations.

4 *transcendent uncertainty*: Perhaps 2020 is too early for this insight: a clinical problem as an expression of nature will illude full understanding. Clinical medicine will focus on evidence that is useful in addressing the pain and suffering experienced by the COVID-19 patient.

5 *nature-change uncertainty*: As a viral condition, COVID-19 can be expected to change.

6 *nature-complexity uncertainty*: As a viral condition, COVID-19 is expected to be complex, despite the hope that manipulating the virus can successfully treat a patient.

7 *value-ambiguity uncertainty*: In the case, the clinical goal to "find a cure and decrease the global health burden and mortality rate" is uncertain because it is unclear what the cure will be and whether it will decrease the global burden and mortality rate.

8 *value-kind uncertainty*: In the case, the clinical goal to continue to treat the patient contrasts (competes?) with providing the patient comfort care. Such value-tensions are typically challenging in medicine today given the ability of medicine to sustain patient lives.

9 *choice uncertainty*: In the case, and given the questionable futility of the treatment, the patient's family chooses in the midst of uncertainty about COVID-19 that the loved ones receive comfort care. I can only imagine that the family struggled with such a decision given the limits of what we knew about COVID-19 at the time.

The bottom line is that there are various levels, kinds, and dimensions of clinical uncertainty in day-to-day clinical decision-making. Given the urgency of a pandemic, such levels, kinds, and dimensions pose challenges to clinicians and patients (and their families) as they needed to work through new clinical evidence, what aspects of an emerging clinical problem is most serious, and what value tensions could be addressed and in what ways during a health care crisis.

Intersectionality of Clinical Uncertainty

Although the prior taxonomy distinguishes levels, kinds, and dimensions of clinical uncertainty, they are not separate and distinct. They deeply intersect. Knowing COVID-19 reflects ways of coming to terms with clinical phenomena and what we single out as worthy of knowing for purposes of diagnosing, predicting, treating, or preventing. For instance, our search to understand COVID-19 is framed by an evaluative goal to treat patients who suffer, which is limited by what we know and the choices we make within particular contexts. The nature of COVID-19 reflects accepted clinical standards for knowing and treating a disease based on collective professional and patient efforts to manage it. For instance, what we call

COVID-19, at any specific time, is a reflection of how we understand it and how we single it out as a legitimate focus of treatment in the clinic, the profession, and society. What and how we value in medicine reflects what clinical objects are signaled out and how we come to know them. For instance, our attention to the risks, harms, and costs of COVID-19 fuels our attention to coronaviruses and the promotion of initiatives focused on treating and preventing COVID-19.

Correspondingly, the uncertainties embedded in clinical knowing, the known, and valuing intersect. In the case of COVID-19, uncertainties about how we know COVID-19 impacts uncertainties about what we know about the clinical problem. That is, limits on our methods frame limits on that which we are trying to understand. Alternatively, the changing and complex nature of a clinical problem impacts how we know it. Uncertainties about what we know about COVID-19 impacts uncertainties about the value judgments we make that influence our efforts to develop tests and treatments. Alternatively, uncertainties about how we value or disvalue COVID-19 impacts uncertainties about how we know COVID-19 and in turn how we develop health protocols and policies during the pandemic.

The point is that, while the epistemological, ontological, and axiological levels, kinds, and dimensions of clinical uncertainty can be distinguished for purposes of education, they intersect in critical ways. Psychologist Chiara Pomare and colleagues (2019) make this point when they propose a revised model of uncertainty in complex health care settings in response to Han et al. (2011). While their model addresses managing uncertainties in health care systems, we'll apply these lessons to managing uncertainties in clinical decision-making. Pomare et al. propose "a reflexive archetype that recognizes different issues of uncertainty while establishing that these are often interrelated in health care systems" (2019, 176). For instance, uncertainties about institutional processes and structures during the pandemic can lead to uncertainty regarding what choices to make in managing a clinical problem. Think here of how confusing public health protocols (e.g., on masking and social distancing) undermined clinical judgment and care during the pandemic (Ho, 2020). Correspondingly, fixed public health protocols (e.g., the isolation of COVID-19 patients) as responses to uncertainty undermined more flexible clinical judgment, the ability to change course after documenting the toll of patient isolation, and subsequently care during the pandemic (Leap, 2023). Further, different issues of clinical uncertainty are interrelated in health care systems in part because there are stakeholders with different identities, experience, and powers. A patient's experience of uncertainty, for instance, will likely differ from a clinician's experience. A minority patient's experience of uncertainty, for instance, will likely differ from a privileged patient's experience. For

Pomare et al., an interrelated account of clinical uncertainty contributes to "more informed and reflective decision-making" (2019, 176). Think of the importance ombudsmen played during the pandemic in rallying on behalf of nursing home clients who were transferred back and forth between nursing homes and hospitals (Chang et al., 2023).

In terms of the proposed taxonomy, and taking Pomare et al. further, consider the relations between and among the levels, dimensions, and kinds of clinical uncertainty we have developed so far.

Figure 5.1 depicts an expanded and intersectional account of clinical uncertainty. It is expanded to include ontological and axiological considerations along with the epistemological ones that are prominent in the clinical literature. It is intersectional because the levels, kinds, and dimensions of clinical uncertainty are seen to stand not in binary opposition (e.g., the uncertainties of knowing vs. the known, knowing vs. valuing, the known vs. valuing), but in nonbinary relation (e.g., the uncertainties of knowing and the known, knowing and valuing, the known and valuing). For instance, uncertainty regarding the probability of a clinical event (e.g., death from COVID-19) raises uncertainty regarding the changing nature of the clinical problem (e.g., COVID-19) which raises uncertainty regarding the choices we make or ought to make regarding a clinical

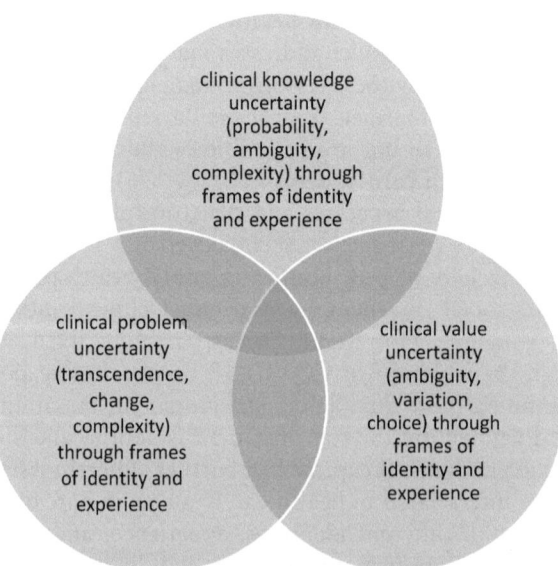

Figure 5.1 Intersectionality of clinical uncertainty.

course of action (e.g., to recommend this treatment as opposed to another treatment). For another example, the complexity of our clinical knowledge of a clinical problem (e.g., COVID-19) raises uncertainties about what and how to value when making an ethical decision in medicine. How we know, what we know, and what and how we value in clinical medicine under conditions of uncertainty intersect and shape each other.

Further, how we know, what we know, and what and how we value in clinical medicine under conditions of uncertainty intersect and shape each other in ways that define and sustain clinical practice. Given that clinical practice entails patients with particular identities and protocols that reflect dominant standards of thought and action, the intersectionality among knowing, the known, and what is valued is framed by the identities and experiences of the stakeholders (patients and clinicians) and in turn frames them. This means that different degrees of inclusion and disclusion, privilege and oppression, and power and weakness will emerge. Think here of who was most served during the pandemic (e.g., those who were able to isolate in the comforts of their own home with the resources that were needed) and who was left behind (e.g., those who were abandoned by our social safety nets). The point is that acknowledging and perhaps understanding how intersecting systems and identities operate to produce privilege and oppression, or care systems that work and those that leave others behind, provides guidance into how we might disrupt the unjust status quo by addressing and dismantling the inequities it perpetuates.

This way of thinking called "intersectionality" arises out of the work of feminists over the last few decades (Crenshaw, 1989, 1991). It focuses on how knowing, the known, and valuing are situated and shape knowledge, practice, reality and our choice situations (Sherwin, 2006, 5; Cutter, 2012). Kimberlé Williams Crenshaw (1989) introduced the idea of "intersectionality" to demonstrate how such dimensions frame the lives of Black women and the discrimination and oppression that they experience in terms of their interlocking racial and gendered identities. According to feminist sociologist Kathy Davis, intersectionality has two distinct characteristics. First, intersectionality unpacks "effects of race, class, and gender on women's identities, experience, and struggles for empowerment" (Davis, 2008, 71). It shows how identities of difference (in terms of, e.g., age, sex/gender, race/ethnicity, caregiver role/the care for role, class/economic status, social role/empowerment, ability/disability, religion/spirituality) impact experiences of power and discrimination. In medicine, such experiences occur in clinical care and its access. Second, intersectionality assists in deconstructing the "binary opposition and universalism inherent in the modernist paradigms of Western philosophy and science" (Davis, 2008, 71). In terms of this project, an intersectional account of clinical problems reveals how assumptions and claims about how we know, what we know, and what and how we value generate, shape, and maintain dimensions of identity, difference, and need. It reveals explicit, as well as implicit, binary oppositions and universal paradigms found in clinical medicine that guide (and hinder) care in clinical medicine.

Davis' second point about binary opposition and universalism resonates in this inquiry. COVID-19 is a term medicine uses for observed signs of the lung and associated symptoms reported by a patient. Granted, in the twenty-first century, it is also a term that refers to the asymptomatically ill who do not experience symptoms, but who test positive for COVID-19. Either way, COVID-19 is an evolving notion that provides structure and significance to clinical reality and patient narratives (e.g., difficulty breathing, fatigue, and coughing) within the context of clinical specialties (infectious disease, immunology, neurology, epidemiology). In talking about COVID-19, then, one must identify the particular community of clinicians and patients to which one makes reference. Is one talking about an account of COVID-19 offered in 2020 or 2023? Is one talking about the Delta or Omicron variant and, if so, which subtype? Is one referring to a 40- or 70-year-old patient, a patient with comorbidities, a patient who works in a service industry with large public exposure, or a patient who just traveled from a country on the World Health Organization watch list for COVID-19? Is one referring to a privileged patient who has the resources to purchase expensive medical care or a patient who lacks regular access to health care, lives in overcrowded housing, or one who cannot advocate for herself? Is one referring to a key worker versus a teleworker? The point is that context matters for the diagnosis, prognosis, and treatment of COVID-19. COVID-19 is not one universal clinical problem (Rosén et al., 2022); it is a heterogeneous clinical condition understood within particular contexts of epistemic, ontological, and evaluative uncertainties.

Davis' first point about the social dimensions of identity receives further attention in Chapter 7, but I'll make a few comments here. Social dimensions of identity, difference, and need conveyed by how we know and value COVID-19 generate, shape, and maintain how COVID-19 is understood and treated. As we all well know, the pandemic has unearthed a number of challenges medicine has had in caring for members of particular populations. The U.S. Centers for Disease Control and Prevention (CDC) reports this:

> [t]he COVID-19 pandemic has brought social and racial injustice and inequity to the forefront of public health. It has highlighted that health equity is still not a reality as COVID-19 has unequally affected many racial and ethnic minority groups, putting them more at risk of getting sick and dying from COVID-19.
>
> (2021e)

As the CDC reports, "[n]egative experiences are common to many people within these groups, and some social determinants of health have historically prevented them from having fair opportunities for economic, physical, and emotional health" (2021e). Here social determinants are wide-ranging. Economic insecurity, access to clean water and nutritious food, safe shelter and workplace, access to waste management, exposure to toxins, intergenerational trauma, and access to education are distributed along lines of social power and contribute to clinical problems (Berkhout and Richardson, 2020). A lesson from the pandemic is striking: as of August 2022, and in a total of over 84 million cases of COVID-19, race/ethnicity was known for 65% or over 55 million cases. In a total of over 880,000 deaths, race/ethnicity was known for 85%, or over 750,000 (Hill and Artiga, 2022). And among these were many of our elders (Freed et al., 2022). When did it register that certain populations were being affected more than others during the pandemic? Were there concerted attempts to consider the intersections among demographic populations or "multiply positioned community members" (Berkhout and Richardson, 2020, 2; also see Sasser et al., 2021) in assessing the toll of the pandemic? Were there practices that we could have rethought to protect members of such populations? Did we experience pandemics as opposed to a pandemic (Maestripieri, 2021)? In what ways were our clinical uncertainties not addressed so that we could have altered our clinical perceptions and actions during the pandemic(s)? An intersectional approach to clinical uncertainty calls us to consider and manage the uncertainties we have about clinical knowledge, clinical problems, and clinical evaluations within the framework of identities of difference and power.

Need for Guidance on How to Manage Clinical Uncertainty

The levels, kinds, and dimensions draw attention to the pervasive and notable ways clinical uncertainty frames clinical knowledge, clinical problems, and the values that guide clinical action. Although such levels, kinds, and dimensions can be distinguished, they interrelate in important ways. They interrelate to reveal the impact contexts and key assumptions have in knowing and valuing a clinical problem. This interrelation can create challenges for clinical decision-makers, especially when managing clinical uncertainty. On this note, it is appropriate to consider how we can manage clinical uncertainty, the topic of Chapter 6.

6 Managing Clinical Uncertainty

A Practical Focus

So far, the analysis has been focused on the theoretical character of clinical uncertainty. This chapter considers the more practical challenge of managing uncertainty in clinical decision-making, with special focus on clinical decisions about COVID-19. It reviews prominent literature on how to manage clinical uncertainty in terms of managing disease uncertainties, health care professional uncertainties, patient and family-centered uncertainties, and health care system uncertainties. It then offers a taxonomy of managing clinical uncertainties in terms of epistemological, ontological, and axiological levels. For instance, when faced with clinical uncertainty, one can clarify risk assessments and trade-offs, remind oneself that clinical uncertainty is not a failure, and reflect on which clinical values are shared and which ones are at odds. It also addresses the moral virtues of managing clinical uncertainty, namely, humility, flexibility, and courage.

Suggestions on Managing Clinical Uncertainty

There are a number of suggestions regarding managing clinical uncertainty during the COVID-19 pandemic found in the clinical literature. A Google search of the phrase "managing clinical uncertainty" provides a host of articles on various topics. These include managing clinical uncertainty with the use of decision-making aids (Bae, 2014), communicating clinical uncertainty (e.g., Santhosh et al., 2019), and role-playing situations involving clinical uncertainty (e.g., Wolpaw et al., 2009). There are also discussions about managing clinical uncertainty in the context of special populations (e.g., intensive care units [Dunlop and Schwartzstein, 2020], oncology [Mishel, 1981], and pediatrics [Brennan, 2003]).

Let's consider an account of managing uncertainty during the COVID-19 pandemic by physician Jonathan Koffman and his colleagues (2020). In their account of managing clinical uncertainty developed for clinicians,

DOI: 10.4324/9781032620978-6

they seek "to acknowledge its presence and, where possible, to work more effectively and efficiently alongside it to improve patient and family care at a critical moment in their lives" (Koffman et al., 2020, 211). They divide their recommendations into managing disease uncertainties, health professional uncertainties, patient and family-centered uncertainties, and health care system uncertainties. These suggestions complement the analysis found in this project in that they distinguish managing clinical problem (e.g., disease) uncertainty from clinical knowledge (e.g., professional, patient) uncertainty. Let's consider each of these sets of suggestions.

Regarding managing disease uncertainties, Koffmann et al. advise that we (1) "[d]evelop and evolve guidance" (2020, 212) based on expert opinion and evidence-based medicine to inform important areas of clinical practice, (2) "[c]ount" (2020, 212) observations and evidence, (3) develop "shared learning for health care professionals … to inform best practices" (2020, 212), (4) "build databases that can inform clinical care … with an awareness of limitations" (2020, 212) in the data that is collected, and (5) develop "robust clinical trials" (2020, 212). In the context of COVID-19, we witnessed significant efforts to develop guidance as evidence emerged, gather data, develop shared learning among health care professionals, build databases, and develop robust clinical trials. We also witnessed significant challenges with gathering and evolving evidence as it emerged, getting information and resources out in a way that was effective and efficient, and rethinking how to use the resources in new and creative ways. Having the data during a pandemic is one thing; messaging it well is another. Expecting shared learning communities during a pandemic is one thing; creating practices to build community is another. Having resources during a pandemic is one thing; distributing them well is another.

Regarding managing professional uncertainties: Koffmann et al. advise that we (1) "[a]dmit uncertainty is not a failing" (2020, 213), (2) pay attention to "burnout, moral distress, and moral injury" (2020, 213), (3) "[r]ehearse situations of uncertainty individually and collectively" (2020, 213), (4) "[b]e aware of cognitive biases" (2020, 213), and (5) teach uncertainty to health care professionals through "clinical learning, case-based approaches and training in health systems" (2020, 213). In the case of COVID-19, we witnessed significant efforts to roll information out and design protocols that erred on minimizing the risks of infection to clinicians and patients. We experienced significant challenges in managing clinical uncertainty as we erred on the side of protocols that failed to take into consideration unintended side effects on vulnerable populations (Leap, 2023). We experienced significant challenges in addressing change in messaging when needed, addressing burnout and moral distress among health care workers and acknowledging cognitive bias when it comes to who was more impacted by the spread of SARS-CoV-2.

Regarding managing patient and family-centered uncertainties, Koffmann et al. advise that clinicians (1) treat "[p]atient/families as allies" (2020, 213); (2) recognize that "[h]elp is available with difficult conversations" (2020, 213); (3) "[b]e imaginative" (2020, 213); and (4) be empathetic by "seeing the world as the patient sees it" (2020, 213), "understanding the patient's current feelings" (2020, 213), "being non-judgmental" (2020, 213), and "communicating that one understands" (2020, 213). In the case of COVID-19, we witnessed significant efforts to design protocols in the hospital that protected clinicians and patients. We experienced significant challenges in being creative about enhancing interactions among clinicians, patients, and their families. Restricting visitations by social workers, mental health counselors, and pastoral counselors contributed to a level of social isolation and lack of patient care that has left its mark today (Jackson, 2020).

Another focus in Koffmann et al.'s analysis is on managing health institutional uncertainties, a topic that this inquiry does not treat at length. Koffmann et al. recommend that we (1) attend to the "four 'S' " (2020, 212), or four key domains that are relevant to alleviate health care system uncertainties associated with COVID-19: stuff, staff, space, and systems. They also recommend that we (2) "[p]repare new systems more specific to the pandemic" (2020, 212) by reconfiguring sites and services, protecting patients and staff, allowing easier delineation between COVID-19 and non-COVID-19 related diseases, and forming "triage and 'reverse triage' pathways based on those most likely to benefit in the event demand for medical services significantly outweigh supply" (2020, 212). Here it is important to (3) "[l]earn from uncertainty" (2020, 212) to uncover "preventable variation, erratic practices, safety errors or near misses, or areas on which new knowledge-new processes are valuable" (2020, 212). This is an important point because the clinician–patient relationship operates within a broader social system. Koffman et al. (2020) rightly remind us that stuff, staff, space, and systems matter as we manage clinical uncertainties. In the case of COVID-19, one is reminded about how resource restrictions (e.g., PPEs), staff challenges (e.g., burnout, resignations), space constraints (e.g., hospital beds and rooms for pandemic and non-pandemic patients), and system failures (e.g., involving the distribution of medical resources) challenged the delivery of care during the pandemic. In our haste to be "right" or "certain," we lost focus too many times on the need to manage clinical uncertainty.

While Koffman et al. give us many things to consider, there are some things missing. This concerns managing value or moral uncertainty. For more on managing moral uncertainty, consider the moving analysis shared by physician Trisha Greenhalgh. Reflecting upon her own experience with the death of her mother, Mary Greenhalgh, from COVID-19, her own health risk factors as a cancer survivor, and the risk factors of her loved ones, Greenhalgh shares with us insight into how to manage moral uncertainties in clinical decision-making. As Greenhalgh reports, her mother was briefly admitted to a hospital following a fall in late December 2020 and during the time that COVID-19 raged in England. Soon after, her mother developed a fever, tested positive for COVID-19, and was readmitted to the hospital. As Greenhalgh reports, her mom became sicker, more distressed, more confused, and closer to death. Add on to this that earlier, her mom expressed that "she did not wish to be placed in a ventilator or admitted to the intensive care unit" (2021, 2644). As was the case with most hospitals at this time during the pandemic, the hospital was overwhelmed with COVID-19 patients, few patients and staff had been vaccinated, the staff was overwhelmed (if not homesick themselves), and the hospital had adopted a no-visitor policy, except for end-of-life compassionate care. Greenhalgh found herself in a dilemma faced by many of us during the pandemic: whether or not to visit her dying mother in the hospital at the height of the pandemic and given the risk of infecting herself and her loved ones.

Greenhalgh reflects on her dilemma through the lens of major ethical frameworks (i.e., goal-based or consequential, duty-based or deontological, and practical rationality and involving emotions). More specifically, she explores the moral uncertainties raised when faced with having to weigh her filial piety and kinship duties to her mother against the wider commitments to the community (2021, 2646). She concludes that managing her moral uncertainty requires a "reflexive" approach, one that is not reducible to any one ethical framework and that moves beyond the confines of each. In the end, Greenhalgh decides not to visit her mother in order to protect her husband from undue harm. As she put it, "the chance that someone would die as a consequence of my actions was low, but if that did happen, it would be very, very wrong" (2021, 2646). She considers the filial duty she has to her mother as well as the emotions that guide her decision. In the end, her adult son, a doctor who had been vaccinated against COVID-19, visited her mother and sat by her side during her final hours. Her mother passed away at the age of 94.

There is much to be grateful for Greenhalgh's self-reflective contextual inquiry is an approach not often found in the clinical and bioethical literature. I'll focus on three lessons that we can consider and save the topic of how to navigate between and among ethical considerations in a reflexive or reflective manner for Chapter 8. The first is working within constraints of value ambiguity, in this case the tensions among traditions of moral reasoning (e.g., consequential, duty-based, practical rationality) (2021, 2644–2646). Here Greenhalgh shows us how to be "reflexive about the temptation to cherry pick" moral theories "to suit the decision we favour"

(2021, 2646). A second lesson concerns how to submit the moral traditions in which one lives to analysis as one considers each within the context of one's moral situation. Here Greenhalgh models how to "maximise doing right and minimize doing wrong" (2021, 2646) as well as one's "filial duties and kinship ties" (2021, 2646) "against the wider commitments to the community" (2021, 2646). A third lesson concerns the importance and inevitability of choice in medicine. Greenhalgh chooses because she must choose, not in terms of "a dispassionate appraisal of empirical facts or formal value hierarchies" (2021, 2646), but in light of "emotional responses, this time directed towards my husband" (2021, 2646).

I'll add one more lesson about managing moral uncertainty to the account that Greenhalgh shares with us. Greenhalgh's focus is on how she navigated her own moral deliberations about visiting a loved one during the COVID-19 pandemic. At first blush, one could read this as an internal exercise of an individual moral agent that is meant to give guidance to other moral agents. This contrasts with a focus on the collective, social, organizational, institutional, and cultural contexts in which a moral agent operates. A focus on the latter would lead us to call for changes in our institutional structures that support managing moral decisions, particularly under conditions of uncertainty (Grady, 2022). This leads us to call for shared learning communities and educational initiatives supported by health care institutions. This leads us to change institution processes through, for instance, alternative ways family and friends could visit their loved ones in the hospital during a pandemic. Think here of the use of acrylic or plexiglass barriers in hospital settings and alternative meeting points (e.g., outside space) so that patients and families could meet (Gan, 2020). In hindsight, there were other options we could have considered earlier in the pandemic (e.g., increased home health and telemedicine options).

A Taxonomy of Managing Clinical Uncertainty

Taken together, Koffmann et al. (2020) and Greenhalgh (2021) give us much to think about regarding managing clinical uncertainty. Let's apply these lessons within the context of the taxonomy that we have developed in this project (see Table 6.1).

The general lesson here is that recognizing clinical uncertainty is not a failure. It is part and parcel of clinical knowledge, clinical nature, and clinical values. One will not be able *simply* to discover, by appeal to factual issues alone, what diagnoses, prognoses, treatments, and preventions of COVID-19 are indicated and what diagnoses and treatments are appropriate. Rather, one also creates them through a rich array of clinical facts, explanations, and values (Cutter, 2003; Sassower and Cutter, 2007).

Table 6.1 A taxonomy of managing clinical uncertainty

Philosophical level	Kind	Dimension	Uncertainty example	Managing uncertainty
Epistemological	Clinical knowledge uncertainty	Probabilistic uncertainty	We are uncertain because clinical knowledge is probabilistic.	Seek to understand or clarify risk assessments and trade-offs. Consider the risk data, evidence, guidelines, and standards of care within the context of shared clinicians and patient (and clinician–patient) learning communities.
		Evidence-ambiguity uncertainty	We are uncertain because clinical knowledge is ambiguous.	Expect clinical ambiguity. Ask about what is unclear, lacking, or at odds regarding the evidence within the context of shared learning communities.
		Evidence-complexity uncertainty	We are uncertain because clinical knowledge is complex.	Expect clinical complexity. Ask about what is complex, and break down complexity in terms of what is known and what is uncertain, and focus on what is known.
Ontological	Clinical problem uncertainty	Transcendent uncertainty	We are uncertain because a clinical problem cannot fully be known.	Admit that one cannot know everything about a clinical problem.
		Nature-change uncertainty	We are uncertain because a clinical problem changes.	Expect clinical problems to change. Pay attention to what changes in the clinical problem and focus on what is alterable.

(Continued)

Table 6.1 (Continued)

Philosophical level	Kind	Dimension	Uncertainty example	Managing uncertainty
Axiological	Clinical value uncertainty	Nature-complexity uncertainty	We are uncertain because a clinical problem is complex.	Expect clinical problems to be complex. Pay attention to the conditional factors and outcomes of a clinical problem and focus on what is alterable.
		Value-ambiguity uncertainty	We are uncertain because clinical values are ambiguous.	Expect ambiguity in clinical values. Reflect on what is unclear, lacking, or at odds regarding the values that guide decision-making within the context of shared learning communities.
		Value-kind uncertainty	We are uncertain because clinical values vary.	Expect that clinical values can vary in kinds (e.g., welfare vs. autonomy). Reflect on which values are shared and which differ, and their implications in proposed clinical resolutions and action plans. Work with what clinical values are shared.
		Choice uncertainty	We are uncertain because we choose to be uncertain or others choose that we are uncertain.	Expect choice uncertainty. Reflect on the extent to which one chooses uncertainty and the extent to which others choose that one is uncertain. Take action to change such uncertainty, when needed.

Acknowledging such realities sheds light on the clinical decisions one makes and the implications of one's decisions. Acknowledging such realities goes hand-in-hand with acknowledging the role of clinical uncertainty in one's decisions. Acknowledging such realities may lend some relief—relief from frantically searching for answers that are not and never will be forthcoming.

And then there is this: after one has managed one's uncertainties and made decisions in light of available clinical observations, tests, and/or pharmaceutical interventions, one will need to come to terms with the reality that one has made a series of decisions based on clinical information, a set of values, external constraints, and an array of other considerations—and these considerations have led one to where one is at present. Of course, there could have been more tests, information, communication, and conversations. There could be more technologies, treatments, and time. There could be less pressure, confusion, anxiety, and fear. There could be different policies and laws in the profession and society. One chooses among options, manages trade-offs, and accepts a clinical course of action in light of what is known, what is available, what is advised, what works, and what is valued at a given time. That's the best one can do in medicine in a world of clinical uncertainty.

Part of the challenge is that there is not one way to manage uncertainty. As Han says, there "is no single, universal, 'right' answer to the question of how to manage uncertainty in medicine or any realm of human life" (2021, 91). He goes on:

> [d]etermining the appropriate management of uncertainty is ... a complex task that requires more than deciding whether uncertainty should be cured or palliated, reduced or endured. It requires justifying this decision with reference to high-level moral goals—that is, the ultimate be goals that specify how people ought to live with uncertainty.
>
> (2021, 89–90)

In the case of COVID-19, determining the level, kind, and dimension of clinical uncertainty is a start, and then managing it for purposes of moving toward such ultimate goals follows. This may entail coming to terms with the limitations of what is known about the viral condition or its treatments, or addressing the moral ambiguities that present in the case when faced with very sick patients.

What might these ultimate moral goals be? For Han, "the ultimate moral goal of uncertainty management must consist of UT [uncertainty tolerance] in a broader sense: *the capacity to achieve an optimal, adaptive balance of responses to uncertainty*" (2021, 91, my italics; also see Simpkin and Schwatzstein, 2016). Reminiscent of Aristotle's teaching (1941), such a balance "depends ... on each individual's own needs, values, and goals, as well as the particulars of the situations" (Han, 2021, 91). In a higher-level sense of metacognitive balance, UT "consists of three more specific goals—moral virtues that enable UT and represent ideal character traits or dispositions that human beings aspire to" (Han, 2021, 94). For Han, these include humility, flexibility, and courage. Humility is a "disposition to be aware of one's limitations in knowledge" (Han, 2021, 95) and "is a necessary precondition for uncertainty and all subsequent efforts to manage it" (Han, 2021, 95). Flexibility allows "individuals to move across their diverse, conflicting psychological responses to uncertainty and to adjust their mix—that is, to find an adaptive balance of responses in a given situation" (Han, 2021, 95). Courage allows "individuals to move ahead from the known present to the unknown future, in spite of their uncertainty and their conflicting responses to it, in order to get on with their own lives" (Han, 2021, 96).

I think we can all think of examples when we witnessed clinical humility, flexibility, and courage in medicine during the pandemic. One story that comes to mind occurred in early January 2020 in China during the pandemic. As reported, Chinese ophthalmologist Dr. Li Wenliang was reprimanded by the Chinese government for messages he posted in a chat group that were false claims that misled the public. He warned fellow doctors about a mysterious form of SARS his patient contracted at the South Island Chinese Seafood and Fruit Market. Li was detained and questioned by the police at the Wuhan Municipal Bureau for Public Safety because he disrupted social order. He returned to work after signing nondisclosure statements and reportedly treated a female patient for glaucoma who had been invested with SARS-CoV-2 from her daughter. Soon after, Li became infected with SARS-CoV-2 and died on February 7, 2020 (Lei and Renzong, 2020).

The Li case also highlights clinical arrogance, stubbornness, and fear. We all have stories of our own experiences with health care leaders who claimed to know things about COVID-19 when they didn't, refused to change in light of new evidence about COVID-19, and engaged in fearmongering in order to resist change in how we cared for COVID-19 patients (Mandavilli, 2021). Bioethicist Anita Ho recounts her experience in 2020 as she traveled between the U.S. and China. When in Hong Kong, she recalls the solidarity individuals displayed in wearing masks in order to prevent against the spread of SARS-CoV-2. Public discussion focused on how to wear masks properly and where to acquire them. When Ho returned to the U.S., messages were different. The CDC "recommended only symptomatic people, front-line clinicians, and family care-givers for sick relatives wear masks" (Ho, 2020, 7th P).

Given that little was known about the spread of SARS-CoV-2, why did the U.S. err on a side of minimal response in 2020? Ho suggests that "[a] commitment to epistemic humility based on limited or evolving evidence is warranted" (2020, 12th P).

The message is that acknowledging uncertainty is essential for success in clinical medicine. It is essential for epistemic, ontological, and evaluative humility, flexibility, and courage, especially during a health care crisis. Physician Jerome Groopman puts it this way: "Does acknowledging uncertainty undermine a patient's sense of hope and confidence in the physician and the proposed therapy?" (2007, 155). No it does not. He goes on:

> Paradoxically, taking uncertainty into account can enhance a physician's therapeutic effectiveness, because it demonstrates his [or her] honesty, his [or her] willingness to be more engaged with his [or her] patients, his [or her] commitment to the reality of the situation rather than resorting to evasion, half-truth, and even lies.
>
> (Groopman, 2007, 155)

Learning to be comfortable working within a world of uncertainty "makes it easier for the doctor to change course if the first strategy fails, to keep trying" (Groopman, 2007, 155). Such is in keeping with clinical knowledge and the nature of clinical problems and clinical evaluation. In this way, uncertainty "is essential for success" (Groopman, 2007, 155) because it requires us to tailor our methods of knowing to that which can be known and to allow for open dialogue and discussion in medicine about clinical matters. It allows clinical knowers and doers to be open to new possibilities and ways of thinking about the detection, prediction, and treatment of disease.

One might say that developing a capacity to achieve an optimal adaptive balance of responses to uncertainty is a tall order during a pandemic. Showing humility during a pandemic appears weak. Being flexible during a pandemic risks being seen as indecisive. Showing courage during a pandemic may appear too bold. Such responses may miss the point: managing clinical uncertainty is a perquisite in good clinical medicine, whether or not this is during a pandemic. There is no choice among those in clinical practice but to face it. Not facing it is a denial of the character of clinical knowledge, clinical nature, and the role of values in clinical decision-making. Facing it allows one to be prepared for the time when decisions must be made at a faster pace in the context of a new emerging disease and during a time when the distribution of resources becomes a matter of life and death.

Need to Think Through the Ethical Implications of Clinical Uncertainty

Our prior discussion focuses on how one can manage uncertainty in clinical decision-making. Managing uncertainty in clinical decision-making is not simply a prerequisite for coming to terms with the limits of knowing and treating clinical problems, it is an ethical responsibility. It is an ethical responsibility because the promotion of welfare, respect for person, fair and equitable distributive distribution of resources, and care in medicine can only be achieved if one manages uncertainty in medicine. It is to this topic that the discussion next turns.

7 Our Ethical Duty to Manage Clinical Uncertainty

Prominent Duties in Medicine

Identifying and acting upon uncertainty in clinical decision-making is not simply an academic or practical exercise; it is an ethical or moral one. Identifying and responding to uncertainty in clinical decision-making highlights the ethical responsibilities that come with making decisions in the clinical setting. As physician Ronald Domen says, "[a]n ethical analysis of ambiguity [or uncertainty] makes it clear that the educators and learners must be aware of their responsibility to treat each other with respect and as human beings and not as objects" (2016, 1; also see Tannert et al., 2007). Think about it this way. Health care professionals and patients make decisions about clinical options. There are observations and tests to interpret. There are decisions regarding therapeutic options. These decisions are nested in prominent ethical duties in medicine to promote welfare, to respect rights, to advance social justice, and to care for each other. Given that these decisions entail uncertainty, they are to be carefully made. Failure to manage uncertainty in clinical decision-making can lead to unnecessary harms, violations of rights, unfair distribution of resources, and the undermining of clinical care.

This chapter shows how managing clinical uncertainty is an ethical duty. It reviews prominent ethical duties in medicine, namely, to advance welfare, respect rights, promote justice, and care for one another in clinical relationships. It shows that managing clinical uncertainty is a prerequisite to satisfy such ethical duties. Failure to manage uncertainty in clinical decision-making can lead to unnecessary harms, violations of rights, unfair distribution of resources, and the undermining of clinical care. It further shows that managing clinical uncertainty calls for reflective equilibrium and intersectional thinking. Reflective equilibrium entails a state of balance or coherence among a set of values arrived at by deliberative mutual adjustment among moral appeals. An intersectional approach refers to a way of thinking and practice that situates

DOI: 10.4324/9781032620978-7

how systems of inequity based on identities of difference (e.g., sex/ gender, race/ethnicity, ability/disability, class/economic status, religion/ spirituality, age) come about and define experience. Reflective equilibrium and intersectional thinking incorporate a personalized dimension to moral deliberation that complements personalized medicine, a clinical approach that addresses clinical uncertainty. Given that managing clinical uncertainty is a prerequisite to satisfying prominent ethical duties in medicine, it follows that there is an ethical duty to manage clinical uncertainty.

Welfare, Rights, Justice, and Care

Ethics is a major branch of axiology and the one that receives the most attention in philosophy, especially in biomedical ethics. It is the study of right and wrong, and good and bad, applied to the actions and character of individuals, families, institutions, and society. Generally in ethics, we apply the terms "right" and "good" to those actions and qualities that foster the interests or stakes of individuals, communities, and society. We apply the terms "wrong" and "bad" to those actions and qualities that impair the interests of individuals, communities, and society (Sassower and Cutter, 2007). There are many ways to talk about ethical interests, and they vary in terms of language (e.g., principles, values) and methodology (consequentialism, deontology, virtue ethics). Today, there are four prominent ways to talk about ethical or moral interests in medicine: welfare, rights, justice, and care. Let's consider these ethical interests in a general sense and how managing clinical uncertainty is critical for the achievement of each of these ethical principles in clinical medicine.

Welfare and Risk Assessment

A first way to talk about interests in ethics is in terms of welfare. Synonyms here include well-being, happiness, prosperity, health, and the good. As philosopher John Stuart Mill says, "The creed which accepts as the foundation of morals 'utility' or the 'greatest happiness principle' holds that actions are right in proportion as they tend to promote happiness; wrong as they tend to produce the reverse of happiness" (1979 [1861], 7). In this tradition, that which advances welfare is labeled "right" or "good" and moral agents should pursue those consequences. In the case of COVID-19, the development of a vaccine is good because it advances the welfare (e.g., health, survival) of those who may contract COVID-19. That which impairs or harms welfare is labeled "wrong" or "bad," and moral agents should not pursue such consequences. For example, in developing a vaccine, it is incumbent to ensure that the vaccine does more good (e.g., proper respiratory function) than harm (e.g., pain and suffering) to those who receive it.

Of course, welfare can be individual or collective. An individual's welfare is measured in terms of bodily, mental, and social well-being. In medicine, it is measured by the results of patient history, screens, tests, and responses to treatment. An individual also has a public welfare as a member of a community and a being whose health depends on others. During the pandemic, we all became familiar with different accounts of viral transmission (e.g., airborne or aerosol, surface or survival) and prevention (e.g., social distancing, isolation, quarantine, vaccines, boosters) promoted by those in authority. We all received a lesson on herd immunity, where herd immunity is resistance to the spread of an infectious disease within a population that is based on preexisting immunity of a population of individuals as a result of previous infection or vaccination. We all received a lesson on the role of comorbidities and the environment in individual and public health, as we became aware of who was more vulnerable to COVID-19.

Welfare in medicine is typically measured by determining and weighing benefits and harms, or what is called "risk assessment." Here, risk assessment "involves the analysis and evaluation of probabilities of negative outcome, especially harms" (Beauchamp and Childress, 2019, 244; also see Gigerenzer, 2002). "Risk" refers to a "possible future harm" (Beauchamp and Childress, 2019, 244) and "harm" refers to a "setback to interests, particularly in life, health, and welfare" (Beauchamp and Childress, 2019, 244). Harm is a complex notion that involves considerations ranging from physical harm to psychological harm. Statements such as "*minimal risk, reasonable risk*, and *high risk* usually refer to the chance of a harm's occurrence—its probability—but often also to the severity of the harm if it occurs—its magnitude" (Beauchamp and Childress, 2019, 244, my italics). In medicine, there is a long-standing moral obligation to minimize patient harm. There are some harms that involve low probability and low magnitude of harm. One thinks here of taking a recommended dose of ibuprofen for a fever. Others involve high probability and high magnitude of harm. One thinks here of an experimental treatment for COVID-19. Others are some combination thereof. Harms that involve high probability and high magnitude are typically of great concern in medicine. Harms that involve low probability and low magnitude are typically of less concern in medicine. Because of variations in the probability and magnitude of the harms brought about by disease and its treatments, medicine has devoted much attention to the gathering of risk assessment data for medical interventions of particular diseases.

Risk assessments and the development of protocols to respond to them are not simply a scientific exercise; they are moral ones. Bioethicists Christoff Tannert and his colleagues argue that

> when it comes to decisions that affect people's lives and health—the regulation of potentially harmful substances or diagnostic tests to predict an individual's propensity to develop a severe disease—carrying out research to diminish uncertainty and, consequently risks can become an ethical duty.
>
> (2007, 892)

Epistemologically speaking, "[u]ncertainties challenge the central claim of science: that all problems are presumed to be solvable by research" (Tannert et al., 2007, 895). Morally speaking, while "[u]ncertainty itself has no ethical quality" in and of itself because it is an inherent attribute of the situation, "uncertainty can trigger ethically adjusted behavior that aims to avoid dangers and diminishes risks" (Tannert et al., 2007, 892).

It follows that managing uncertainty in medicine in a context of an emerging clinical condition is an ethical duty in order to promote the welfare of those in medicine. In the case of COVID-19, screenings and diagnostic tests are developed with the intention to reduce false positives and false negatives. Treatments and preventive measures are developed to maximize benefits and minimize harm to the patient and the public. If we do not acknowledge the clinical uncertainties entailed therein, we cannot develop safe screenings and tests for patients and safe practices for health care workers. If not, we cannot treat patients well with an eye toward minimizing harms and maximizing benefits. If not, we cannot develop effective preventive measures for clinical conditions. Acknowledging clinical uncertainty is necessary in order to advance a patient's welfare in medicine.

Rights and Informed Consent

A second way to talk about ethical interests is in terms of a *right* or rights. In moral philosophy, a right is a claim or entitlement to be treated a certain way because of one's status. Synonyms here are autonomy, dignity, liberty, or freedom. The notion of right has a long history and is rooted in the claim that a moral agent is autonomous and thus worthy of respect. As philosopher Immanuel Kant said, "Act so that you treat humanity, whether in your own person or in that of another, always as an end and never as a means only" (1985 [1785], 47). One way that we treat a person as a "end" is to acknowledge his, her, or their "right." For instance, some argue that patients have a "right" to be treated equitably, and therefore securing informed consent from a competent patient ensures that patients are treated equitably. Respect for rights promotes interests because it allows moral agents to choose to pursue what they value. For instance, the practice of securing informed consent from a COVID-19 patient in need of treatment is based on the moral duty to respect the rights of the patient. Denial of rights damages someone's interest because denial does not allow moral agents to pursue their individual values and social freedoms. On this view, denial of rights should be prevented. For instance, not securing informed consent from a competent COVID-19 patient undermines his, her, or their dignity, and therefore should be prohibited.

Informed consent is a complex notion and practice. According to Beauchamp and Childress, there are seven components of informed consent:

I   Threshold elements (preconditions)
    1 Competence (to understand and decide)
    2 Voluntariness (in deciding)
II Information elements
    3 Disclosure (of material information)
    4 Recommendation (of a plan)
    5 Understanding (of 3 and 4)
III Consent elements
    6 Decision (in favor of a plan)
    7 Authorization (of the chosen plan) (Beauchamp and Childress, 2019, 122)

Applied to our discussion, informed consent in COVID-19 care entails (1) a patient's ability to understand her condition and decide her course of action, (2) a patient's voluntariness or freedom to decide her course of action, (3) the provision of relevant or material COVID-19 information, (4) a health care professional's recommendation of a relevant plan of treatment, (5) a patient's ability to understand incoming information and to have relevant beliefs about the nature and consequences of the proposed treatment plan, (6) a patient's ability to decide in favor of or against a treatment plan, and (7) a patient's ability to authorize a course of action for COVID-19 care and proceed accordingly.

Despite our best efforts, there are numerous challenges with securing informed consent during a pandemic. (1) A patient's ability to understand and decide, (2) a patient's freedom to do so without constraints, (3) the availability of relevant and clear material information, (4) the availability of a relevant and clear plan of action, (5) a patient's ability to understand and process 3 and 4, (6) a patient's ability to make a decision in a particular situation, and (7) the patient's ability to authorize and follow through in a plan of action are each fraught with uncertainty. This is the case because clinical diagnoses, prognoses, treatments, and preventive measures are limited, open to change, and evaluative, especially during a pandemic involving a newly emerging clinical condition that can have serious consequences. It follows that health care professionals will find themselves in a situation of securing "less-than-informed" and "less-than-free" informed consent from a COVID-19 patient. A COVID-19 patient will be deciding and authorizing a plan of action on incomplete information about the diagnosis, prognosis, treatment, and prevention of COVID-19.

Nevertheless, the practice of informed consent as an expression of respect for patient autonomy is not doomed. A start is to recognize that managing clinical uncertainty is a prerequisite for respecting autonomy and securing informed consent. Physician Ronald E. Domen argues that "an understanding of the ethics of ambiguity [uncertainty] is important to fostering the virtue of respect and before a patient-centered approach can be established and be successful" (2016, 2). If one is unable to address clinical uncertainties, then one will not be able to develop effective learning in medicine and provide patient-centered care. Managing clinical uncertainty leads to a number of positive measures in medicine, which includes improved personal well-being, effective mentorship, a culture of respect imbedded throughout the institution, meaningful learning, and meaningful physician–patient relationships and patient-centered care (Domen, 2016, 6). Think about it this way: false informed consent is not informed consent. Conveying and discussing clinical uncertainty, recognizing the uncertainties of clinical information and what is known, creating space to promote the ability of decision-makers, and envisioning the informed consent process as a fluid one are called for (The Conversation Project, 2022). Perhaps it is time to confront this more directly in the informed consent literature and revise clinical practices to give time for discussion about what is known and what is uncertain about what one is agreeing to. Acknowledging clinical uncertainty is necessary in order to respect patient autonomy.

Justice and Health Equity

A third way to talk about ethical interests is in terms of *justice*. The ethical principle of justice guides our thinking about what is fair, equitable, and appropriate in light of what is due to persons. Synonyms here are inclusion, equality, equity, fairness, and right. The term "justice" comes from the Latin root "*justus*," meaning "just" or "right." Justice is one of the oldest moral principles dating back to the Ancient Greek philosopher Aristotle (384–322 B.C.E.) (1941). As Aristotle says in the *Nicomachean Ethics*, "the just, then, is the lawful and the fair, the unjust the unlawful and the unfair" (1941, 1129a, 34–35). Common to all theories of justice is Aristotle's mandate to "treat equals equally," and "treat like cases alike." Justice promotes moral interests because it seeks a fair or equitable distribution of benefits and burdens. For instance, allocating ventilators for COVID-19 patients on the basis of who will clinically benefit most is the just thing to do. Undermining justice should be avoided because it erodes moral order in medicine in that it violates standards of fairness, equity, and inclusion in caring for patients. Allocating ventilators only to those who can pay is unjust because it turns a caring profession into one in which only those who can pay can participate. While there may be some free market exchanges in medicine that can be justified (e.g., voluntary aesthetic treatment services), treatment for conditions that are not chosen (e.g., a disease brought about by a transmissible virus) requires a different account of justice.

Justice

> refers to fair, equitable, and appropriate distribution of benefits and burdens determined by norms that structure the terms of social cooperation. Its scope includes policies that allot diverse benefits and burdens such as property, resources, taxation, privileges, and opportunities, food distribution, jury service, and service as a research subject.
>
> (Beauchamp and Childress, 2019, 268)

The call for justice in medicine highlights the moral imperative that no persons should receive social benefits on the basis of undeserved advantageous properties because no persons are responsible for having these properties. No persons should be denied social benefits on the basis of undeserved disadvantageous properties because they also are not responsible for these properties (Beauchamp and Childress, 2019, 282–286). The goal is health equity, or a state in which everyone has a fair opportunity to attain their optimal health regardless of identities of difference (e.g., gender, race, economic class, age, and disability). In the case of COVID-19, properties, such as a contagious virus and vulnerable health status, are not chosen by individuals and thus do not provide grounds for morally accepted denial of or discrimination in health care. It follows that access to beds, ventilators, treatment, and care should not be denied.

Nevertheless, justice is a challenging principle to uphold in a world of limited resources. Consider a number of ways in which health care resources can be allocated:

1 To each person according to rules and actions that maximize *social utility* (utilitarianism)

2 To each person a maximum of liberty and property resulting from the exercise of liberty rights and participation in fair *free-market exchanges* (libertarianism)

3 To each person according to principles of fair distribution derived from *conceptions of the good* developed in moral communities (communitarianism)

4 To each person an equal measure of liberty and *equal access to the goods in life* that every rational person values (egalitarianism)

5 To each person the means necessary for the *exercise of capabilities* essential for a flourishing life (capability theories)

6 To each person the means necessary for the realization of core *elements of well-being* (well-being theories) (Beauchamp and Childress, 2019, 271)

Consider an example of each distribution model. (1) Following their availability, COVID-19 vaccinations were distributed on the basis of social utility. Front-line workers were the first to receive them. (2) Private health care remained available in the U.S. throughout the pandemic for those choosing to pay for additional care. (3) The goal was to distribute PPEs according to conceptions of the good, although we all know that that was a challenge. (4) "Free" COVID-19 antigen tests were distributed equally, insofar as one requested them through government websites. (5 and 6) Free COVID-19 testing clinics were set up across the nation in accordance with advancing the capabilities and well-being of those in need.

Alternatively, we can think of violations of the principle of justice during the pandemic. Isolating patients to the point of undermining their mental and physical health can be seen to violate social utility and equal access to the goods of life, especially when particular populations of patients (e.g., the elderly, the economically disenfranchised) were most affected (Lowrey, 2021; Ruble, 2021). Access to private health care during a public health crisis is justified on grounds of free-market exchanges, but is problematic when resources (e.g., PPEs, vaccines, boosters) are necessary for the health and good of all during a pandemic. Distributing resources in large metropolitan cities, when service workers often live in outlying areas, illustrates a failure to think through what constitutes equitable access and efforts to advance moral capability and well-being.

The point is that managing clinical uncertainty is a prerequisite for promoting justice. Without a sense of the clinical uncertainties of a clinical problem, efforts at social justice fail. As mentioned in Chapter 5, the Centers for Disease Control and Prevention (CDC) (2021b) early on in the pandemic recognized that older adults and people with severe underlying conditions (or comorbidities) were at higher risk for developing serious complications from COVID-19. It described COVID-19 as extremely contagious, presenting in patients from vulnerable populations as sudden and unpredictable respiratory and multisystem failure, leading to high mortality in patients 65 and older and sudden death in others with compromised immune systems, and presenting with worse outcomes in those with comorbidities. This by itself is not grounds for a claim about unjust practices. The problem is that populations of vulnerable individuals were treated differently during the pandemic. According to Avik Roy, in May of 2020 and at the height of the pandemic and the Delta variant, 2.1 million Americans, representing 0.62% of the U.S. populations, resided in nursing homes and assisted-living facilities. In the 43 states that reported such figures in 2020, 42% of all COVID-19 deaths took place in nursing homes and assisted-living facilities (Roy, 2020).

There's so much more to say about how the elderly were treated during the pandemic. The health care system isolated the elderly, transferred them back and forth between their residents and health care facilities, denied them family visitors, restricted counselors and spiritual advisors from visiting patients, and we can go on (Lowrey, 2021). We witnessed the use of refrigerator trucks for dead bodies outside Bellevue Hospital in New York City and the mass grave on Potter's Island in New York and elsewhere (Neilson, 2020; "Pictures of the Year," 2021). We heard about or experienced ourselves restricted funeral and memorial services for COVID-19 patients. As Professor of Health-Care Policy David Grabowski says, "What the hell were we doing?" (cited in Lowrey, 2021, 3rd P). My sentiments, exactly.

In addition to the elderly, members of racial and ethnic populations suffered significantly during the pandemic. The U.S. CDC report this:

> [t]he COVID-19 pandemic has brought social and racial injustice and inequity to the forefront of public health. It has highlighted that health equity is still not a reality as COVID-19 has unequally affected many racial and ethnic minority groups, putting them more at risk of getting sick and dying from COVID-19.
>
> (2021e)

As the CDC reports, "[n]egative experiences are common to many people within these groups, and some social determinants of health have historically prevented them from having fair opportunities for economic, physical, and emotional health" (2021e).

As of August 5, 2022, the CDC reported a total of over 84 million cases of COVID-19, for which race/ethnicity was known for 65%, or over 55 million (Hill and Artiga 2022, 2). It reported a total of over 880,000 deaths, for which race/ethnicity was known for 85% or over 750,000 deaths (Hill and Artiga, 2022, 2). More specifically, American Indian

(AIAN), Hispanic, Native Hawaiian, or Other Pacific (NHOPI), and Black people are more than twice as likely to die from COVID-19 compared to their White counterpart. Note that data reported in 2022 appears to be underestimated as they do not reflect individuals who tested positive on home tests and who did not report findings to their public health agencies. The higher rates of infection and death likely reflect "increased exposure risk due to working, living, and transportation situations, including being more likely to work in jobs that cannot be done remotely, to live in larger households, and to rely on public transportation" (Hill and Artiga, 2022, 6).

Managing clinical uncertainty is a prerequisite for justice in health care. If we do not come to terms with clinical uncertainty, we operate with inaccurate information and practices. If we operate with inaccurate information and practices, we make decisions about social utility, free-market exchanges, conceptions of the good, equitable access to the goods of life, and ways to support the exercise of capabilities and elements of well-being that do not reflect human health needs. They do not reflect human needs because they fail to take into consideration the intersectionality among individual health, the community, the environment, and social systems. For instance, key to achieving health justice is recognizing how food deserts, poor quality education, inadequate housing, and unfair and unhealthy employment practices create and sustain inequitable health outcomes, particularly during a pandemic, play critical roles. Key here is acknowledging what we may not know and what we may not want to know about. Acknowledging clinical uncertainty is necessary for the achievement of health justice, equity, and inclusion in medicine.

Care in Clinical Relationships

A fourth way to talk about ethical interests is in terms of *care*. Moral agents have relationships in which certain expectations and responses arise because of his, her, or their vulnerability or needs. On this perspective, individuals are seen to be in unequal relationships in which one is more vulnerable and receives care. Individuals who are more vulnerable deserve considerations in proportion to their disclusionary status, and situational factors determine how to promote the interests of those in the relationship. Actions that advance care are morally worthy because they recognize and respond to an agent's vulnerabilities or needs. For instance, the elderly, as vulnerable members of our society, qualify for preferential treatment in medicine during a pandemic that disproportionally affects them. Preferential treatment might include early vaccinations, preferential entry into a hospital, or financial assistance. But it is not simply about utilitarian preference; it is about what constitutes compassionate care, where

compassionate care entails a state of sympathy for another, and especially the vulnerable, and taking actions to assist, when needed. Actions that do not advance care are morally problematic because they fail to recognize and respond to an agent's vulnerabilities or needs. Isolating elderly patients for extended periods of time without attending to the effects of such isolation on their well-being can be seen to be a violation of proper care for members of a vulnerable population.

In *Caring: A Feminine Approach to Ethics and Moral Education*, philosopher of education Nel Noddings (1984) argues for the moral preferability of a care perspective in ethics that orients moral agents to focus on the needs of others in relational contexts rather than on abstract, rational moral principles (e.g., welfare, rights, justice). Noddings starts with the view that care relationships (involving the "one-caring" and the one "cared for") are basic to human existence and consciousness. They involve a natural human affective response and the memory of being cared for as a subject, as opposed to an object. They generate moral obligations that are contextually applied, as opposed to ones that are generated from universal moral principles. In the case of COVID-19, prioritizing care to members of vulnerable populations and those who are in relationships of care (e.g., parents, teachers, clinicians) reflects this. Recall that in the early phase of the pandemic, lists were developed about who first should receive the vaccines. While first responders, clinicians, and the elderly were on top of the list, service workers (e.g., grocers, bus drivers) were not. This led to a significant rise in COVID-19 cases and deaths among service workers (Cotofan et al., 2021), many of whom were from racial and minority groups. It is no wonder, then, that members of racial and minority groups expressed distrust of medicine when it rolled out further vaccines and boosters (The Commonwealth Fund, 2021).

Care ethics considers moral judgments to be rooted in everyday, situated, social practices. Care ethics entails duties to maintain human relationships by contextualizing and promoting the well-being of caregivers and care-receivers within social systems of power. Special attention is given to acts of compassion for the vulnerable, or those most dependent on others. Here, compassion is a state of sympathy for another, and especially the vulnerable, and taking actions to assist in appropriate ways. In these contexts, emotions play a key role in guiding us toward someone or something, with a level of degree depending on the relationship and the need. As Martha Nussbaum (2003) reminds us, we appraise a moral situation with and through our emotions and relationships. In the case of COVID-19, recall Greenhalgh's moral dilemma about whether to visit her dying mother in the hospital during the pandemic. As Greenhalgh tells us, "[b]ringing emotion into the theoretical frame means that subjectivity, gut feelings and kinship and friendship ties can be embraced and theorized rather than rejected" (2021, 2645). Guided by her emotions when she arrived at the hospital with her husband by her side, she reports:

> I felt a wave of powerful emotions—this time towards the man who had walked in step with me for 34 years and was committed to supporting whichever choice I made. If I entered the hospital to visit our loved one, I would be consciously and avoidably placing another loved one at risk … . I felt shame towards myself and a growing protective instinct towards my partner.
>
> (2021, 2646)

As she shares: "I could not bring myself to go in. Instead of holding my dying mother's hand, I grasped my husband's" (2021, 2646). Nussbaum's message is clear: "emotions do *moral work*: they embody judgements about values. We feel emotional about something we care about. Emotions, so often dismissed as irrational, nonsensical and to be controlled and suppressed, are actually evaluative in nature and should be engaged with" (Nussbaum, 2003, cited in Greenhalgh, 2021, 2646). Far from needing to suppress our emotions in order to appraise a situation, we appraise the situation with and through our emotions.

One of the challenges in making space for emotions in moral decision-making is that emotions can be uncertain. They can be uncertain in terms of their kind (e.g., joy or sadness, love or hate), their direction (e.g., positive or negative), and their degree (e.g., strong or weak). With these variations comes uncertainty. Nevertheless, managing clinical uncertainty is a prerequisite for the achievement of care in medicine. Managing the clinical uncertainties that are rooted in everyday, situated, clinical practice takes time, patience, and awareness of what is known and what is uncertain. It takes honesty, a willingness to be engaged in the care relation, a commitment to what is occurring in the life of a health care professional and patient, and an openness to change in action plans, when needed. If we do not take into consideration clinical uncertainty in how we care for each other in medicine, then the care relation will be static, objectifying, or one-size-fits-all, as opposed to fluid, responsive to an individual as a person, or in tune with what is needed at a given time. Acknowledging clinical uncertainty is necessary in order to deliver compassionate care in medicine.

Managing Clinical Uncertainty as a Precursor to Satisfying Clinical Duties

The prior discussion details ethical implications of managing clinical uncertainty in order to advance welfare, respect rights, promote social justice, and care for others in medicine. It considers the need to acknowledge clinical uncertainty in order to act ethically in medicine. It correlates a kind of clinical uncertainty with an accepted ethical duty in medicine and its material or practical expression, thereby illustrating how addressing clinical uncertainty is necessary for the achievement of prominent ethical duties in medicine. If we do not recognize and manage clinical uncertainty, there are a number of ethical implications: we cannot develop evidence-based risk assessments and thereby promote patient best interest and minimize patient harm. We cannot develop proper informed consent processes and thereby respect patient and clinician in their decision-making. We cannot distribute clinical resources fairly and thereby promote health equity. We cannot tailor clinical tests and treatments to the individual patient and thereby care properly for patients. If we do not manage clinical uncertainty, we cannot fulfill prominent duties in medicine.

Consider the following abbreviated schema (see Table 7.1).

A failure to take clinical uncertainty can lead to absolutism and unwavering policies in medicine that have implications for advancing a patient's best interest, respecting a patient's autonomy, promoting health equity, and caring for patients. I recall the day during the pandemic when the elder care ethics committee on which I serve read "Growing Old," by journalist Anne Lowrey (2021). In it, Lowrey investigates how the elderly were faring during the pandemic. She shares part of her interview with physician David Grabowski, professor of health care policy at Harvard Medical School:

> When we look back on this [our clinical treatment of the elderly during the pandemic] in the years to come, I imagine there's going to be a lot of Monday-morning quarterbacking around whether it was a good idea to blockade older adults in their nursing home rooms for eight, nine, 10 months out of the year, without letting them have access to their families.
>
> (Lowrey, 2021, 3rd P)

Committee members grappled with this problem, well attuned to local, regional, and state policies around health care visitations. Grabowski's response to such practices resonated with us: "I think we're going to look back and say, 'What the hell were we doing?'" (Lowrey, 2021, 3rd P).

The schema shared in Table 7.1 sheds further light on the case of restricting visitations to the elderly in health care facilities during the pandemic. At the time Lowrey wrote her essay, people over the age of 85 were "630 times as likely to die of COVID-19 as people in their 20s" (Lowrey, 2021, 4th P) and "40 percent of coronavirus death" occurred "in institutions housing fewer than 1 percent of Americans" (Lowrey,

Table 7.1 Ethical implications of managing clinical uncertainty

Ethical duty	Material expression	Role of clinical uncertainty	COVID-19 example
Advance welfare	Risk assessment	Determining risks in a population and applying the data to an individual patient	How do I understand the risks of the recommended treatments in my own case of COVID-19? What are the trade-offs in choosing the recommended care?
Respect rights or autonomy	Informed consent	Securing free and informed consent from a patient in the context of limited information and constraints	What do I need to know in order to make the best decision about COVID-19 treatment? What information is most relevant and what is uncertain?
Promote social justice	Just allocation of clinical resources	Allocating clinical resources in a fair, equitable, and inclusive way	Are COVID-19 resources being distributed in a way to advance health equity? In what ways do I participate in practices that contribute to health inequity (e.g., ordering too many or too little tests, developing absolutist or no health policies)?
Care for each other in medicine	Care relationships	Prioritizing care in medicine	Does our health care institution foster proper care for COVID-19 patients, to those most vulnerable, and to an individual patient?

2021, 4th P). In terms of best interest, we failed the elderly. In terms of patient autonomy, social justice, and care, we failed them. We failed them because we developed absolutist policies in health care that were based on incomplete information, a limited view of COVID-19, and a value system that failed to take into consideration a vulnerable population during the pandemic. We failed to take seriously the role of clinical uncertainty in decision-making, which if we did would have allowed us to be attuned to changing information about COVID-19, be imaginative and fluid with proposed policies, and care for members of vulnerable populations.

Reflective Equilibrium and Intersectional Thinking

Managing clinical uncertainty is crucial in our efforts to promote welfare, rights, social justice, and care in medicine. While these duties can be distinguished, as they were in the prior chapter, they interrelate. Acting in favor of a patient's interest and respecting a patient's right often go hand-in-hand. Informed consent documents typically reflect a commitment to advance a patient's welfare and respect patient autonomy. There will be situations in which 3w76 one duty is more prominent than another. Respecting the right of a competent patient to refuse treatment is a duty in medicine, even when a clinician holds that treatment would be beneficial. There will be situations in which the particular duties clash. A clinician's duty to protect a patient's welfare by imposing isolation policies during a pandemic can override a patient's request to see family members in the hospital. The intersections between and among ethical duties are made all the more challenging when faced with clinical uncertainties. Given this, it will be critical to think through how to manage the intersections among ethical duties in medicine, especially in cases of conflict.

Bioethicists Tom Beauchamp and James Childress provide guidance on managing differing, if not competing, ethical duties. Drawing from philosopher John Rawls (1971) and his account of "reflective equilibrium," Beauchamp and Childress instruct that

> [w]henever some normative feature in a person's or a group's prevailing structure of moral views conflicts with one or more of their considered judgments (a contingent conflict), they must modify something in their viewpoint and strive to achieve equilibrium and overall coherence.
>
> (2019, 440)

Reflective equilibrium begins with a body of beliefs that are acceptable initially without argumentative support. These beliefs occur at all levels of moral thinking, from more concrete considerations (e.g., practical, psychological, and I would add in agreement with care ethicists, emotional) through normative values and principles (e.g., welfare vs. rights) to metaethical or theoretical conceptions (e.g., secular vs. faith-based duties). As beliefs are developed and conflicts between and among beliefs emerge, individuals "must modify something in their viewpoint in order to achieve equilibrium" (Beauchamp and Childress, 2019, 440).

In the case of COVID-19, and applying Greenhalgh's case study in my own life, my filial duty (e.g., to visit my loved one in a hospital) may compete with my duty to follow institutional and legal policies (e.g., to comply with a no-visitor policy). The goal of reflective equilibrium "is to match, prune, and adjust considered judgments, their specifications, and other beliefs to render them coherent" (Beauchamp and Childress, 2019, 440–441). For instance, perhaps it would be possible to set up visitations in which the patient and family members were properly distanced and fitted with PPEs in a ventilated environment, while following institutional and legal policies. Individuals "then test the resultant guides to action to see if they yield incoherent results" (Beauchamp and Childress, 2019, 441). If it does, then the actions must be readjusted. For instance, if a hospital is not set up for alternative visitations that are safe for all involved, this approach does not lead to coherent results. Asking someone else in the family who works at the hospital to visit my mother on my behalf may lead to coherent results. In thinking through ethical issues in medicine and taking a stance, it will be important to attend to specifying the ethical theories, principles, and values as they operate and intersect within specific contexts.

By "specifying," Beauchamp and Childress mean "narrowing the scope of the norms" (2019, 17). Narrowing the scope of the norm involves "spelling out where, when, why, how, by what means, to whom, or by whom the action is to be done or avoided" (Beauchamp and Childress, 2019, 17). Here reflective equilibrium involves a process of advancing, considering, and revising claims with regard to the moral problem under consideration and in light of the multiple, and perhaps conflicting, values, principles, or duties that are at stake. It involves, as well, attention to the uncertainties that frame and permeate how we know, what is known, and how and what moral agents value. As we now know, clinical knowledge, that which we know, and the values we bring to our clinical decisions are to some extent uncertain. Visiting loved ones in the hospital virtually may not provide the comfort that we seek to provide to our loved ones. Our loved ones may not welcome this alternative approach. We may have questions about institutional and legal policies regarding the efficacy of social isolation during the pandemic, and the harms that result from such isolation. Such reflections are to be expected and encouraged, for perfection is not the goal. As Beauchamp and Childress say, "[p]ersons involved in rendering norms coherent should not expect an end to this process of revision that provides a complete normative account" (2019, 441). The process is "a continuous work in progress—a relentless process of improving moral norms and increasing coherence" (Beauchamp and Childress, 2019, 441). The process entails continuous attention to the tensions and conflicts between and among moral norms, seeking to develop options and alternatives in order to achieve better coherence. And, I would add, the process entails continuous attention to the role of uncertainty in clinical decision-making.

Consider a more general case and one that involves the moral maxim "respect the COVID-19 patient's right to refuse vaccination." Contemporary biomedical ethics places great emphasis on this maxim because patients are seen to be worthy of respect as individual decision-makers. Upon reflection, the moral maxim is not absolute, but intersects with other moral maxims such as "do not harm the patient," "benefit the patient," "benefit the patient's family," "follow proper standards in clinical practice," "follow the rules of the hospital," "protect the public," and so on. While the moral maxim "respect the COVID-19 patient's right to refuse vaccination" is an acceptable starting premise, we are left with a range of options about how to specify this rule and balance it against other norms. For instance, the moral maxim to respect the COVID-19 patient's right to refuse vaccination is balanced with the moral maxim to minimize harm to the patient, to benefit the patient, to secure justice in health care, and to care for the patient. In the case of respecting a COVID-19 patient's right, attention is given to promoting the welfare, rights, justice, and care in medicine. Compromises may have to take place, and when they do, it will be important to be clear on what is being compromised and in what ways in order to reach the best solution. This is what was going on when institutions and governments required individuals to be vaccinated in order to travel or work, and yet proposed processes for opting out of COVID-19 requirements for medical and religious reason. We found ourselves, during a pandemic, having to weigh rights with the welfare of clinicians and patient within a public health crisis. In addition, it will be important to remain open to change and new deliberations, not as a sign of weakness, but rather as an indication that we can know more and do better in a world of uncertainty. And we can change course if needed, which will be important in delivering the best medical care that is available at any given time.

The intersections in reflective equilibrium remind us that our ethical duties do not always fit together coherently with no residual incoherences or conflicts. As Beauchamp and Childress tell us, "[t]he trimming, repair, and reshaping of beliefs will need to occur repeatedly in response to new situations of conflicting norms" (Beauchamp and Childress, 2019, 442).

This is especially the case in the context of clinical uncertainty. Part of our efforts in reflective equilibrium is devoted to matching, pruning, and adjusting considered moral judgments, their specifications, and additional values that enter into our deliberations. Part of our efforts is devoted to clarifying how we know, what we know, and how and what we value—with constant reminders of their limitations. In the case of COVID-19, matching, pruning, and adjusting the values of advancing welfare during a pandemic, respecting rights, promoting social justice, and caring for others receive high priority, even when compromises have to be made. Again, perfection is not and cannot be the goal. The process of reflective equilibrium in clinical decision-making under uncertainty is a process, a process of advancing, considering, and revising claims with regard to the problem under consideration and in light of the multiple, perhaps conflicting, values, principles, and duties that are at stake. This takes humility, flexibility, and courage (Han, 2021): the humility to be aware of limits, the flexibility to change when needed, and the course to stand up to what is right and good.

Done well, reflective equilibrium will be able to disrupt the unjust status quo in medicine if it also attends to the assumptions and claims that frame "status quo" clinical knowledge, clinical problems, and clinical values. As feminist philosopher Nancy Tuana said years ago,

> Cognitive authority is determined by many factors, including the character of a speaker, her or his intellectual capacity, his or her reasonableness, and so on—criteria that feminists have demonstrated to be imbued with the prejudices of sexism, anthrocentrism, racism, classism, ageism, and ableism.
>
> (Tuana, 2006, 13)

Applied to the discussion at hand, reflective equilibrium as an intersectional practice in biomedical ethics can provide a lens to consider the identities and unique structural barriers individuals face. Identities of difference in terms of age, sex/gender, race/ethnicity, caregiver role/a cared for role, and many others frame clinical problems. Here, the "and" is important. Consider age as a criterion in triaging COVID-19 patients. For an intersectional standpoint, "age is not the only thing that makes a person benefit less from a scarce medical resource during a pandemic. Other social identities play a major role in the health status of older individuals, and of the population in general" (Rueda, 2021, 91). Examples here are comorbidities, economic status, and lifestyle factors. An intersectional approach takes seriously the intersections and interactions among numerous contributing factors in one's health status and seeks to "disaggregate data to study the differentiated effects that COVID-19 has had on mortality and morbidity" within the elderly population (Rueda, 2021, 91).

Further, reflective equilibrium and intersection thinking are key components of evidence-based personalized medicine. Contemporary medicine entails a focus on evidence for its findings, coupled with how the evidence relates to the individual patient. Evidence provides empirically verifiable findings that change with new knowledge. Personalized medicine recognizes that there is not a "one-size-fits all" approach to diagnosis, prognosis, treatment, and prevention. Individual patients with so-called similar clinical problems have different genetic, physiological, and environmental components (National Human Genome Research Institute, 2023). Such differences guide decisions about testing, treatment, and prevention. One can only hope that personalized medicine can assist in helping us understand important differences in COVID-19 among patients (Zhou et al., 2021), and especially long COVID. Reflective equilibrium and intersectional thinking incorporate a personalized dimension to moral deliberation that complements personalized medicine.

Need for Further Reflection on Managing Moral Distress

The prior discussion details the ethical implications of managing clinical uncertainty in terms of prominent ethical duties, namely, advancing welfare, respecting rights, promoting social justice, and caring for others. Navigating between and among ethical duties requires reflective equilibrium. Although the prominent ethical duties have been separated in this chapter, they typically work together in an intersectional way. This is especially the case when managing clinical uncertainty. There is no doubt that this can be a challenge, especially during a public health crisis. Those who are making such decisions may experience moral distress that may result in moral fatigue, moral injury, moral betrayal, moral guilt, moral suffering, moral overload, moral resignation, moral burnout, or moral nihilism. In keeping with this theme, Chapter 8 takes a look at managing moral distress and building moral resilience.

8 Managing Moral Distress and Building Moral Resilience

Pandemic Stress

Managing clinical uncertainty has been particularly stressful during the COVID-19 pandemic. The spread of COVID-19 around the world, the evolving nature of SARS-CoV-2, the speed in which clinical information has changed during the pandemic, the severity of the disease condition for members of particular populations, and the health care delivery obstacles that occurred during the pandemic have not been easy for any of us. We have had to manage new clinical information about an emerging virus and its resulting clinical condition, implement new therapeutic and preventive responses, and act in accordance with accepted moral and legal duties in medicine at a fast pace and in light of grave consequences. One of the topics that has received notable attention during the pandemic is how patients and clinicians have been faced with challenges in managing moral distress in clinical decision-making.

This chapter takes a closer look at the challenge of managing moral distress in the context of clinical uncertainty with an eye toward building moral resilience. Managing clinical uncertainty has been particularly stressful during the COVID-19 pandemic. The spread of COVID-19 around the world, the evolving nature of SARS-CoV-2, the speed in which clinical information has changed during the pandemic, the severity of the disease condition for members of particular populations, and the health care delivery obstacles that occurred during the pandemic have not been easy for clinicians and patients. Clinicians and patients have had to manage new clinical information about an emerging virus and its resulting clinical condition, implement new therapeutic and preventive responses, and act in accordance with accepted moral and legal duties in medicine at a fast pace and in light of grave consequences. Given this, coupled with the claim that clinicians and patients have an ethical duty to manage clinical uncertainty, it is important to think about ways to manage moral distress and build moral resilience in the health care setting.

DOI: 10.4324/9781032620978-8

Recognizing Moral Distress

The topic of moral distress received much attention in medicine during the pandemic. According to physician Donald Pathman and his colleagues, "Weighted to reflect all surveyed clinicians, 28.4% reported no moral distress related to work during the pandemic, 44.8% reported 'mild' or 'uncomfortable' levels and 26.8% characterised their moral distress as 'distressing', 'intense' or 'worst possible'" (2022, abstract; also see Murthy, 2022). The reasons for moral distress varied.

> The most frequently described types of morally distressing issues encountered were patients not being able to receive the best or needed care, and patients and staff risking infection in the office. Abuse of clinic staff, suffering of patients, suffering of staff and inequities for patients were also morally distressing, as were politics, inequities and injustices within the community. Clinicians who reported instances of inequities for patients and communities and the abuse of staff were more likely to report higher levels of moral distress.
>
> (Pathman et al., 2022, abstract)

According to nurse and clinical ethicist Cynda Hylton Rushton,

> [o]ur understanding of the stress response can shed light on the negative consequence of moral distress. Humans are hardwired to respond to threats. The most primitive part of the brain—the reptilian brain—identifies threats and signals the body to prepare for action through a predictable series of responses: fight, flight, or freeze. Physical threats, along with such psychological threats as anxiety; emotional upheaval; and a sense that one's goals, values, identity, and (arguably) integrity are in danger, can automatically activate the body's alarm system and shift the brain into survival mode.
>
> (2017, 13)

More specifically,

> [t]he amygdala and connect brain regions go on to detect significant stimuli, and if fear is present—consciously or unconsciously—negative emotions are activated. These include negative arousal, narrowed and biased attention to potential threats, diminished empathy and interference with prosocial behavior, and reliance on automatic default patterns.
>
> (Rushton, 2017, 12)

When one experiences moral distress, one can deregulate the nervous system and activate emotions such as anger, frustration, disgust, and discouragement (Rushton, 2017, 13). This can lead to a variety of responses, such as moral fatigue, moral injury, moral betrayal, moral guilt, moral suffering, moral overload, moral resignation, moral burnout, and moral nihilism. One can be fatigued and exhausted, physically and psychologically, from the attempts at pursuing one's values and duties. One can feel unempowered, and thereby feel injured, betrayed, or guilty. One can suffer from knowing that one has not lived up to one's values or duties. One can experience moral overload, and thereby not be able to process anything further. One can be resigned to moral apathy or moral nihilism.

The notion of moral distress predates the pandemic. In 1984, philosopher and bioethicist Andrew Jameton introduced us to the notion of "moral distress." He defines it as "the experience of knowing the right thing to do while being in a situation in which it is nearly impossible to do so" (Jameton, 1984, 6). He shares with us some background on the development of this notion.

> My 1984 book, *Nursing Practice: The Ethical Issues*, introduced moral distress as the experience of knowing the right thing to do while being in a situation in which it is nearly impossible to do it. I was responding to students' stories related during classroom discussions of bioethical dilemmas, such as appropriate care for dying patients, limits to life support, and communication and decision making with patients and families.
>
> (Jameton, 2017, 617–618)

Jameton's nursing students recalled situations in which they were required to perform painful procedures when, in their experience, curative efforts were futile. Other situations involved suctioning patients on respirators who had been in intensive care units for weeks, but who would not live to be discharged. Jameton shares what he saw as the limits of bioethical approaches that emphasized cognitive moral reasoning and appeals to abstract moral theories:

> I thought it was important to address the emotional side of moral problems. In so doing, I shared the concerns of educators cultivating the moral development of clinical professionals. Nurses were professionally concerned about the role of emotions in providing compassionate care to patients. And feminist moral theory was foregrounding emotional factors in ethical theories based on care, compassion, and empathy.
>
> (Jameton, 2017, 618)

I agree with Jameton (and Nussbaum and Greenhalgh) that biomedical ethics needs to widen its approach to include the role of emotions in ethical decision-making.

Let's take a closer look at the kinds of moral distress and its connection to clinical uncertainty. According to philosopher and bioethicist Carina Fourie, moral distress refers to a situation in which an agent (1) knows what action is morally correct to take, but (2) cannot take the action because there are constraints or obstacles (3) which prevent the agent from taking the action. Fourie calls this "moral-constraint-distress" (2013, 92). Consider a case in which a clinician knows that it is right to respect a COVID-19 patient's wish to have loved ones by her side, but institutional policies and guidelines in which the clinician works prevent patient visitations from taking place. A clinician is put in the situation of having to follow the policies and guidelines as a requirement for employment, inform the patient's family of them, and live with the implications that follow in defending a set of actions with which the clinician disagrees. In this case, the tension between these options, between advancing public health measures and honoring the wishes of a patient, are at odds. Here, the clinician experiences a clash of values and cannot achieve both values, but rather is constrained in acting according to a particular option.

Along with clinicians, patients experience moral-constraint-distress. Consider a case in which an individual who has been diagnosed with COVID-19 is asked to isolate. Assume that individual is employed on an hourly basis in a service industry, needs to make an income for herself and family, and goes to work despite clinical and public policy advice. An individual in a situation like this can experience moral distress knowing that, while it is best to stay home in order to prevent against the spread of a virus, it is also best to go to work to earn an income in order to feed, clothe, and house the family. The constraint of having to earn an income overrides the values of acting in accordance with what is advised during the pandemic. In this case, moral distress may arise from not having the choice to achieve both values.

According to Fourie, moral distress also refers to a situation in which (1) it is morally uncertain which action to take, (2) an agent does not know how to proceed, and (3) an action is not taken or, if it is, it is unclear whether it is a moral option. Fourie calls this "moral-uncertainty-distress" (2013, 93; also see Fourie, 2017). This is a situation in which a clinician does not know which value option is best, and therefore is unclear about what to recommend to a patient. Whatever action (or nonaction) is taken, the clinician is conflicted. Think of the early days of the pandemic when clinicians recommended treatments that had yet to be sufficiently studied.

Along with clinicians, patients experience moral uncertainty-distress. Think of a situation in which a patient is torn about what is the "right" thing to do. In the early months of the pandemic, when one had flu-like symptoms and home tests were not available, but one needed to shop for essentials, many of us asked about whether we should stay home or risk going out. Many of us in this situation pondered whether we should venture into a health care facility or stay home without reporting our symptoms. Many of us thought about whether we should take loved ones with COVID-19 symptoms to the hospital risking their social isolation or dying alone or keep them at home during the pandemic and far away from hospital facilities.

Building Moral Resilience

A common theme in definitions of moral distress concerns the tension or conflict between one's value judgment about the action that should be taken and the inability to carry out that action because of internal or external reasons. How might one respond? According to Rushton and nurse Kathleen Turner, there is a tool that one can use to sort through situations that involve moral distress. Rushton and Turner call this the 4Rs: (1) recognize the situation for what it is, (2) release yourself from past experience and consider what you can now change, (3) reconsider or reframe an issue or view it in a new way, and (4) restart and move forward in a positive way learning from the prior tools (Rushton and Turner, 2020). Greenhalgh (2021) shows us how this takes place as she recognizes the situation that she found herself in, considers what is in her ability to act on and go forward, reframes the problem in terms of varying ethical positions, and arrives at a conclusion that she appears to be at peace with. Such is the basis of building what is called "moral resilience."

Generally speaking, *resilience* is the ability to recover from serious individual or community-level setbacks. According to Rushton, "[r]esilience is a concept that has been applied in various disciplines and has been used to manage adverse events such as natural disasters, war, and climate change and in business, systems, and other domains" (2016). Resilience is the capacity, over time, to regain a sense of agency. It's the ability to put one foot forward, to see what the next step might be and collect oneself to move in that direction. That doesn't mean that having distress, struggling, and even falling down aren't a part of resilience. The key is that one gets back up and tries another approach that lessens the distress and moves one toward one's goal.

According to Rushton, *moral resilience* "is distinct in its focus on (1) the moral aspects of human experience, (2) the moral complexity of the decisions, obligations, and relationships, and (3) the inevitable moral challenges that ignite conscience, confusion, and moral distress" (2016). Currently, according to Rushton, there is no established evidence base for specific strategies for cultivating moral resilience. Nevertheless, she points to a number of promising possibilities for cultivating moral resilience: (1) foster self-awareness, (2) develop self-regulation capacities, (3) develop ethical competence, (4) speak up with clarity and self-confidence, (5) find meaning in the midst of despair, (6) engage with others, (7) participate in transformational learning, and (8) contribute to a culture of ethical practice (Rushton, 2016, 2018). Put another way, one is advised to (1) foster self-awareness on one's values, (2) develop patience in discerning what is evaluatively disconcerting, (3) become informed about how to talk about ethical matters, (4) practice speaking up, (5) accept that change takes time, (6) build learning communities to discuss cases that raise ethical issue, (7) be open to change, and (8) mentor others in such ethical practices. Taken together, these suggestions also highlight the importance of managing the clinical uncertainties that arise in moral decision-making.

In the context of COVID-19, consider a case (Kayser et al., 2021) in which a 35-year-old man with COVID-19 pneumonia and acute respiratory distress syndrome (ARDS) who suffers from multi-organ failure without evidence of lung recovery. The family insists on continued care while multiple health care teams have advised that further treatment is futile. Members of the health care team have voiced that further treatment would be "torture." As a starting point, Kayser et al. (2021) recommend to health care team members to change the perspective in the case, and consider what the family is experiencing. This helps reformulate the claim that treatment is torture and redirects attention to providing care that would be more comforting to the patient (and family). This approach highlights the role that (7) plays in addressing moral distress. The fact that this health care group gathers together to discuss such matters highlights the role that (1), (2), (3), (4), (5), (6), (8) AND managing clinical uncertainties play in addressing moral distress and building resilience.

There are consequences in not addressing moral distress (Rushton, 2018; Grady, 2022). Not addressing moral distress can lead to mental and physical frustration, disengagement, and burnout are a few examples. Such can take a toll on the health care team and undermine its stability and integrity. These can take a toll on patients and undermine their care. Not addressing moral distress can lead to under-responding to a moral dilemma. Health care professionals can simply not care. Not addressing moral distress can lead to over-responding to a moral dilemma. Health care professionals and patients can become rigid or absolutist. I can't help but think that isolating patients and residents over a long period of time, prohibiting funeral or memorial services, and not permitting pastoral counselors into the hospital to visit with dying patients were rigid or absolutist responses (Jackson, 2020).

Alternatively, moral distress can be beneficial. It might mean that we are paying attention and registering concerns, even when we may not be able to change the situation (Ulrich and Grady, 2019). The outrage that clinicians and patients have expressed about allowing patients to die alone reflects an awareness of a practice that needs attention. It might mean one is formulating a response to an institutional practice that needs to be changed. Bringing concerns about social isolation practices to administration or an ethics committee is a step toward making policy changes. Of course, research is needed to distinguish moral injury or burnout from an opportunity for growth.

Nurse and bioethicist Christine Grady agrees with Jameton and Rushton that it is incumbent in the clinical setting to develop ways to address moral distress and assist health care workers in developing moral resilience. During the COVID-19 pandemic, "[s]tudies show the overall increased rates of depression, anxiety, insomnia, burnout, obsessive-compulsive symptoms, and somatization symptoms in healthcare workers" (Grady, 2022, 57; also see Asken, 2020). Among these reports, "the highest incidence of anxiety and depression is found in nurses, females, frontline workers, and those with inadequate training or inadequate PPE" (Grady, 2022, 57). This sociocultural observation of the incidences of moral distress leads Grady to suggest that moral distress and moral resilience are not simply *internal* to the moral agent. They are notably *external* to the moral agent. If one wishes to address moral distress and moral resilience, one will then need to pay attention to the ethical climate of clinical units and organizations, and to the "social, organizational, institutional, and cultural" factors at play (Grady, 2022, 58). During the COVID-19 pandemic, for instance, conditions promoting self-care (e.g., reasonable shifts, time-off) along with institutional support (e.g., sufficient staff, resources to care for patients, transparent communication, administrative support, discussion forums, wellness programs) are critical. Longer-term strategies include opportunities for education and mentoring, attention to power differentials and decision-making hierarchies, and policies and structures that support promoting an ethical workplace culture (Grady, 2022, 59).

A Taxonomy of Moral Distress and Resilience

Given that how and what we value is nested in how and what we know in medicine, moral distress is not simply a moral phenomenon, but an epistemic and ontological one nested in social contexts. Putting this discussion of moral distress and moral resilience in a wider frame of discussion about clinical uncertainty, we arrive at a number of suggestions for managing moral distress and building moral resilience. Consider this abbreviated schema (see Table 8.1).

Table 8.1 A taxonomy of managing moral distress and building moral resilience

Philosophical level	Kind	Recognizing moral distress	Building moral resilience
Epistemological Uncertainty	Clinical knowledge uncertainty	Recognize a situation in which (1) it is morally uncertain which action to take, (2) one does not know how to proceed, and (3) an action is not taken or, if it is, it is unclear whether it is a moral option.	Recognize and seek to understand what is known about the data and the clinical standard, along with their ambiguities and complexities.
Ontological uncertainty	Clinical problem uncertainty	Recognize a situation in which one (1) knows what action is morally correct to take, but (2) cannot take the action because there are external constraints or obstacles (3) which prevent one from taking the action.	Recognize and seek to understand the limits, evolving nature, and complexity of the clinical problem and the external constraints of the situation.
Axiological uncertainty	Clinical value uncertainty	Recognize what values are at stake in the decision(s) that are being made. Recognize which value(s) are important and/or have priority. Recognize what values are in conflict or at odd with others.	Recognize the value tensions or conflicts in the situation. Release oneself from past experiences and consider what one can now change. Reconsider or reframe the value issue or view it in a new way. Restart and move forward in a positive way learning from the prior tools. Evaluate the ethical climate of one's clinical unit or system.

While the messages are simple, the task is great. The greater the clinical uncertainty, the greater one can experience moral distress. Further, as we have learned from this inquiry, the kind of clinical uncertainty and their interactions matters, thus leading to divergent morally distressful responses. For instance, ambiguity of clinical evidence in a case of a mild COVID-19 fever differs from ambiguity of clinical evidence in a case of significant respiratory failure. Working with ambiguity of clinical evidence when one has confidence in surviving differs from working with clinical evidence in a context of life versus death. While the former may elicit some level of moral distress about what one ought to do (e.g., stay home or venture out to work), the latter will likely elicit a morally distressful response regarding whether and how to pursue life-saving treatment.

Need for Further Reflection and Action

A focus on clinical uncertainty leads one to consider situations in which we experience moral distress. Managing moral distress entails epistemic, ontological, and evaluative strategies. Such strategies allow one to build moral resilience in the context of differing and competing values. Such are especially important in situations such as a pandemic, when knowledge of an emerging clinical problem is fast-paced, clinical interventions are being developed, and patients are suffering, if not dying. In such contexts, it becomes evident that managing moral distress and building moral resilience are critical tools in clinical decision-making. This is the case not just during a pandemic, but beyond a pandemic. If we start to put all of this together, we arrive at "an ethics of clinical uncertainty," to which Chapter 9 turns.

9 Toward an Ethics of Clinical Uncertainty

Some Summary Reflections

This book explores the ethical implications of managing uncertainty in the diagnosis, prognosis, treatment, and prevention of COVID-19. Uncertainty pervades clinical decision-making during the COVID-19 pandemic in a number of ways. Clinical knowledge of COVID-19 is uncertain because it is probabilistic, ambiguous, and complex. The clinical problem we call COVID-19 is illusive, changing, and complex. The clinical values that frame our understanding and guide our treatment of COVID-19 are ambiguous, varied, and chosen. As a consequence, it is important for clinicians and patients to acknowledge an expanded notion of clinical uncertainty, manage it, and address its ethical implications in the clinical setting in order to maximize welfare, respect rights, foster justice, and care for each other in clinical relationships. To do this, it is critical that the approach to clinical uncertainty be intersectional and acknowledge the multiple ways in which systems of thought, nature, and values impact and are impacted by the identities and experiences of those in the clinical setting. It is also important to learn how to manage clinical uncertainty in order to manage moral distress and build moral resilience. In the end, this project calls for an "ethics of clinical uncertainty."

Proposed well before the pandemic, physician Christof Tannert and his colleagues (2007) raise the need for an ethics of clinical uncertainty. As they say,

> acting in a state of uncertainty can create ethical problems: ignorance caused by rejection of knowledge can lead to danger. However, knowledge can also lead to ethical problems: it can create risks if the exposed person decides to accept the threat, imposes it on another person or accepts that such a threat is imposed.
>
> (2007, 896)

DOI: 10.4324/9781032620978-9

Tannert and his colleagues focus on the need to engage in risk assessment research and argue that "carrying out research to diminish uncertainty and, consequentially, risks can become an ethical duty" (2007, 892). I would say not just "can," but "must." As this investigation shows, uncertainty permeates all aspects of clinical knowledge, clinical nature, and clinical values. It is the norm, and not the exception in clinical medicine. It is not a "pandemic phenomenon" (although the pandemic heightened our experience of it), but rather a medicine-wide one that acknowledges the character of clinical knowledge, clinical problems, and the role values play in knowing a clinical problem. Given this, it is incumbent that clinicians and patients attend to managing clinical uncertainty. Such is an ethical duty, one that promotes welfare, rights, equitable access to services, and care in medicine.

The ethical implications of not recognizing and managing clinical uncertainty in its expanded and intersectional expressions are notable. If we do not recognize and manage clinical uncertainty, we cannot develop evidence-based risk assessments and thereby promote the best interest of patients and clinicians and minimize their harm. We cannot develop proper informed consent processes and thereby respect the autonomy of patients and clinicians in their decision-making. We cannot distribute clinical resources fairly and thereby promote health equity and the fair opportunity to live a healthy life. We cannot tailor clinical tests and treatments to an individual patient and thereby care properly for patients and those who care for patients. In that such ethical duties interplay, we cannot promote each duty without attending to their intersections and interactions in terms of how they impact and are impacted by the identities and experiences of those in a clinical relationship. If we do not manage clinical uncertainty, we cannot come to terms with the nature of clinical knowledge, clinical problems, and clinical evaluation and thereby fulfill prominent ethical duties in medicine.

In managing clinical uncertainty, one can start by asking about what is uncertain about the clinical evidence, the clinical problem, and what ought to be done about the clinical problem. Recognize at the start that one does not know everything, one cannot know everything, and one (or someone) makes choices in the clinical world about what ought to be done. Starting out with such expectations opens up discussions and lends itself to acknowledging clinical trade-offs, respecting clinical decision-makers, being stewards of limited clinical resources, and participating in a clinical partnership in which the goal is to care for an individual patient.

Domen says "an understanding of the ethics of ambiguity [or uncertainty in medicine] is important to fostering the virtue of respect and before a patient-centered approach can be established and be successful" (2016, 2). Drawing on Simone de Beauvoir (1948), he reminds us of the central importance of recognizing, engaging, and validating each other's autonomy in order to be fulfilled in life. As Beauvoir says: "I concern others and they concern me. There we have an irreducible truth" (1948, 72). As we have learned, such an interdependence in medicine entails uncertainty, but allows for the caring profession we call medicine. Practically speaking, Domen suggests a ' "top-down' approach to teaching the importance of, and tolerance for, ambiguity and uncertainty" (2016, 5). More specifically, he calls for institutional leadership to promote educational programs focusing on the role, importance, and tolerance of ambiguity in medicine. Let's face it: changes in medicine typically come from the top, as they do in any hierarchical institution. Developing education programs in ethics that address managing clinical uncertainty is a start. An integration of ethics education with a focus on managing clinical uncertainty will have an impact on patient care, personal satisfaction, medical education, professionalism, and the health care organization (2016, 5; also see Hansson, 2013; Djulbegovic, 2021; Johnson, 2021). It will also be an important step in introducing intersectional thinking in medicine as it provides a lens to consider identities of difference and the unique structural barriers clinicians and health care professionals experience in their lives, including when they are sick.

In drawing this analysis to a close, we can say that an ethics of clinical uncertainty entails seven notable actions, namely, (1) understand clinical uncertainty, (2) manage clinical uncertainty, (3) recognize the ethical implications of managing clinical uncertainty, (4) practice reflective equilibrium in managing clinical uncertainty, (5) recognize moral distress, (6) build moral resilience, and (7) change institutional practices, when possible. In terms of a framework (Table 9.1), consider the following.

When faced with clinical uncertainty, the message is to reflect on the levels, kinds, and dimensions of uncertainty that present, think through best practices for managing them within the context of the situation, remind oneself that not attending to clinical uncertainty has ethical implications, grapple with the value tensions or conflicts that arise, register when one becomes morally distressed, seek to build resilience when faced with moral distress, and recognize the external forces that frame one's decisions and seek to change institutional practices, when needed. Such is in keeping with good ethical practice and the ethical goals of promoting the welfare and rights of moral agents and working toward health equity in which care for each other is a priority.

Personal Notes

As shared in the Preface, as a clinical ethicist and former cancer patient, I have been trying for years to make sense out of how clinical uncertainties

Table 9.1 A taxonomy of an ethics of clinical uncertainty

Components	Strategy	Examples
1. Understand clinical uncertainty	Seek to understand: a. clinical knowledge uncertainty b. clinical problem uncertainty c. clinical value uncertainty	Clarify: a. how one is uncertain b. what is uncertain, and what is beyond one's ability to know c. what values are uncertain or unable to be acted upon
2. Manage clinical uncertainty	Seek to manage: a. clinical knowledge uncertainty b. clinical problem uncertainty c. clinical value uncertainty	Develop strategies: a. to acknowledge the uncertainty of what is known b. to recognize the illusive, changing, and complex character of a clinical problem c. to clarify value similarities and differences, possible resolutions, and action plans
3. Recognize the ethical implications of managing clinical uncertainty	Identify one's duty in medicine to: a. advance welfare b. respect rights c. promote social justice d. care for those in the clinical relationship	Develop strategies to achieve: a. robust risk assessments b. honest informed consent and communication processes c. fair, equitable, and inclusive allocation of clinical resources d. care for those in medicine, and especially the vulnerable
4. Practice reflective equilibrium in managing clinical uncertainty	Pay attention to: a. the intersections among the levels, kinds, and dimensions of clinical uncertainty b. the intersections among prominent ethical duties in medicine c. the identities of difference and unique structural barriers that frame and are framed by (a.) and (b.)	Develop: a. shared learning communities to discuss such intersections b. dialogue with representatives of diverse stakeholders (e.g., clinician, patient, administrator, finance, members of the community) c. listening and learning skills

Table 9.1 (Continued)

Components	Strategy	Examples
5. Recognize moral distress	Pay attention to: a. the moral distress one experiences when one is conflicted about is the right or good action b. the moral distress one experiences when one knows the morally correct action to take, but external constraints make it impossible to pursue the right action	Seek to: a. recognize what values are or seem to be at stake in the decision(s) that are being made b. recognize which value(s) are important and/or have priority c. recognize what values are in conflict or at odd with others
6. Build moral resilience	Seek to: a. sustain or restore integrity in response to moral distress b. learn from moral distress c. make changes in light of moral distress	Seek to: a. recognize the value tensions or conflicts in the situation b. release oneself from past experiences and consider what one can now change c. reframe the value issue or view it in a new way d. restart and move forward in a positive way e. review the ethical climate of one's clinical unit or system
7. Change institutional practices, when possible	Seek to: a. recognize the external forces that frame knowledge, nature, values, and contexts b. evaluate and revise, when needed, systems, processes, and protocols	Take action to: a. evaluate the epistemological, ontological, and ethical climate of clinical units and systems b. develop safe and transparent processes and lines of communication that support external change c. build shared learning communities that focus on needed changes

operate hand-in-hand with clinical evidence and how we can best manage those uncertainties in the context of clinical decision-making (Cutter, 2018). It is in this project, one written during a pandemic, that I have found insights and resolutions to my own questions concerning how to come to terms with uncertainty in clinical decision-making and how to manage it. I started with these questions: (1) What is COVID-19? (2) What brings it about? (3) How do we know it? (4) What are the best clinical treatments or responses? (5) Can COVID-19 be prevented? (5) How do we respond to 1 through 5 in a clinical world of limited information and action? (6) What are the ethical implications of the decisions we make about COVID-19? (7) What forces frame our clinical decisions and in what ways? It occurred to me that responses to each of these questions entailed kinds and degrees of uncertainty. And so this investigation took shape.

Now that I have had time to work through the investigation, I am able to offer a more extensive look at the levels, kinds, and dimensions of clinical uncertainty that have challenged those of us who have had a voice during the pandemic. And, I am able to say something about the ethical tugs that we have experienced during the pandemic. In arriving at an expanded and intersectional account of clinical uncertainty, and in arguing for an ethics of uncertainty, I hope that we can learn something about clinical uncertainty that can frame future practices during and well after a pandemic.

Beyond what appears in the foregoing inquiry, I have a few more thoughts to share. When under the care of a clinician after being diagnosed with a clinical problem, one might ask: (1) How does the population risk data on the clinical problem apply to me? (2) Even though I have signed the informed consent authorizing intervention, what are my options for having my questions answered? (3) What is uncertain about my clinical condition and its recommended treatments? Given this, what decision would you (i.e., the clinician) make if you were in my shoes? Alternatively, a clinician might ask: (1) How does the population risk data apply to my patient? (2) How can I and my staff be available should other questions arise? (3) What uncertainties do you (i.e., the patient) have about your clinical condition and its recommended treatments? Such is in keeping with good practice making decisions with the information that is available at the time in the face of clinical uncertainty. And, finally, for all parties, pause to listen. It's amazing how opening up quiet space and listening allow additional clinical evidence to emerge from patients and clinicians that is critical in guiding the clinical process.

While this inquiry had not focused in detail on how institutions handle clinical uncertainty, I have a few thoughts on the matter based on the experience many of us had during the pandemic as we obtained clinical information from institutional sources (Sopory et al., 2019). One might recall that the two leading public health agencies, the U.S. Centers for

Disease Control and World Health Organization, disagreed in 2021 on the definition of the pandemic, the frequency of asymptomatic symptoms, and the safety of COVID-19 vaccines for pregnant women (Mandavilli, 2021; Pence, 2021). What might we have learned from their mixed messages? Starting from the premises that clinical uncertainty is inevitable and clinical uncertainty is challenging to navigate, institutions might consider the importance of the following: (1) At the start, be transparent of clinical uncertainty. (2) Communicate information about uncertainty clearly, sharing not only what is not known but how decisions are being made in the context of uncertainty. (3) Be consistent in how information about uncertainty is released, using language to designate uncertain claims (e.g., provisional, update) and different means of dissemination that are accessible to others. (4) Coordinate messages about uncertainty between and among experts carefully and transparently so as not to confuse others. (5) Share actions that are taken place in light of uncertain claims clearly, transparently, and in a timely fashion. These are only a few suggestions, but are a start as we move forward from our experiences during the pandemic.

Suggestions for Future Work and Action

A project like this can only do so much. There are a number of topics that deserve further investigation by those interested in clinical uncertainty. These include:

1 the investigation of intersectional accounts of clinical uncertainty in the context of particular specialties in clinical medicine (e.g., pediatrics, oncology, genetics), select populations (e.g., in terms of age, race/ethnicity, sex/gender, economic status, political beliefs, spiritual beliefs), and individual differences (e.g., the focus of personalized medicine): A contextual treatment of clinical uncertainty will focus on particular clinical problems in order to appreciate the nuances of such particularities within specialized contexts and with regard to diverse identities of difference. Such will be in keeping with the theme of this inquiry that there is not one universal taxonomy of clinical uncertainty. There are lots of room for many, with diverse ethical implications in varying clinical practices. Clarifying such expressions will be theoretically and practically important in particular clinical specialties.

2 the development of educational programs for pre-health care undergraduates, health care graduates, postgraduates, clinical practitioners, and patients about clinical uncertainty: Clinicians and patients can benefit from learning about clinical uncertainty. Programs can be developed within the health care curriculum as well as in care facilities and be responsive to different populations of learners. Such

programs can be lodged within philosophy of medicine sequences, complementing bioethical training that is typically available in clinical educational and training programs.

3 the investigation of social factors (e.g., workplace, education, media, politics) that frame clinical uncertainty, moral distress, and moral resilience: A sociology of medicine approach to clinical uncertainty can unveil the intersectional aspects of knowledge, nature, and values within social systems of thought and action. Such systems situate and define the components of clinical uncertainty and more work is needed in this area by clinical researchers.

4 the development of safe institutional policies and practices for educational forums, complaints, and whistle-blowing: Working under conditions of uncertainty can be unnerving and it will be critical to develop processes that create safe spaces for members of communities when they ask questions, raise concerns, or call for action.

5 the development of institutional coordination for sharing information between and among research groups and distributing medical resources in conditions of uncertainty: If anything, the pandemic has brought us face-to-face with the limits of institutions and their ability to coordinate the distribution of health care resources during a health care crisis marked with uncertainty. More work is needed on developing effective and efficient institutional practices during health care crises and beyond.

6 further reflections on what we have learned from our actions during the pandemic: When I sent off my manuscript to a notable press, an editor quickly got back to me to share that the press was concerned about "pandemic fatigue." As one can imagine, I was in disbelief. How could we have gone through what we went through and witnessed so much need to rethink our actions, and not want to continue to reflect? Thus, I encourage the continuation of reflections on the pandemic. We still have much to learn about ourselves, our practices, and our institutions as we grapple with uncertainties during and after the pandemic.

I'll end there, still processing what we have been through. Manage your expectations about the diagnosis, prognosis, treatment, and prevention of clinical problems. Spend some time reflecting on the uncertainty of clinical claims and actions, and make decisions in light of these considerations. Sort out the uncertainties so that multiple lines of inquiry are encouraged. Take care of each other in medicine, and promote each other's welfare and respect each other as persons. Promote a culture in medicine that is equitable and inclusive—not just in words, but in actions as well. And, last but not least, celebrate what clinical providers and researchers do for us, not only during a pandemic, but in other times. They are the ones who stepped up to the plate during a health care crisis and rallied for best practices in medicine, despite the hurdles and constraints. Celebrate patients as well. They are the ones who said "yes" to public health emergency vaccines, treatments that needed more research, quarantine and lockdown protocols that wreaked havoc in their lives, and health care institutional practices that did not always meet their needs and the needs of their families. They are the ones who can tell us that the pandemic was not the great equalizer as some assumed much greater burdens than others. May we learn from our experiences and may we continue to share such lessons well before the next health care crisis.

References

Anesi, George L. 2022. "COVID-19: Epidemiology, Clinical Features, and Prognosis of the Critically Ill Adult." *UpToDate*. August 15. www.uptod ate.com/contents/covid-19-epidemiology-clinical-features-and-prognosis-of-the-critically-ill-adult?search=COVID-19%20Prognosis&source=search_res ult&selectedTitle=1~150&usage_type=default&display_rank=1

Aristotle. 1941. *Nicomachean Ethics*, in *The Basic Works of Aristotle*. Edited and with Introduction by R. McKeon, 935–1112. New York: Random House.

Asken, Michael. 2020. "Now Its Moral Injury: The COVID-19 Pandemic and Moral Distress." *Medical Economics*. April 29. www.medicaleconomics.com/ view/now-it-moral-injury-covid-19-pandemic-and-moral-distress

Babrow, Austin S. et al. 1998. "The Many Meanings of Uncertainty in Illness: Toward a Systematic Accounting." *Health Communications* 10 (1): 1–23.

Bacon, Francis. 1878. *The Works of Francis Bacon*. Cambridge: Hurd and Houghton.

Bae, Jong-Myon. 2014. "The Clinical Decision Analysis Using Decision Tree." *Epidemiological Health*. 36 (October 30): e2014025. doi:10.4178/epih/ e2014025. PMID: 25358466; PMCID: PMC4251295

Bajaj, Simar Singh, and Fatima Cody Stanford. 2021. "Beyond Tuskegee: Vaccine Distrust and Everyday Racism." *The New England Journal of Medicine* 384 (February 4): e12. doi:10.1056/NEJMpv2035827

Banning, Maggi. 2008. "A Review of Clinical Decision-Making." *Journal of Clinical Nursing* 17 (2): 187–195. doi:10.1111/j.1365-2702.2006.01791.x

Barbey, Aron K. et al. 2014. "Distributed Neural System for Emotional Intelligence Revealed by Lesion Mapping." *Social, Cognitive, and Affective Neuroscience* 9 (3): 265–272.

Bean, William Bennet (ed.). 1950. *Sir William Osler: Aphorisms from his Bedside Teachings and Writings*. New York: Henry Schuman.

Beauchamp, Tom L., and James F. Childress. 2019. *Principles of Biomedical Ethics*. 8th ed. New York: Oxford University Press.

Beauvoir, Simone de. 1948. *The Ethics of Ambiguity*. Translated by B. Frechtman. New York: Philosophical Library.

Berkhout, Suze G., and Lisa Richardson. 2020. "Identity, Politics, and the Pandemic: Why Is COVID-19 a Disaster for Feminism(s)." *History and*

Philosophy of the Life Sciences 42 (4): 1–6 https://philpapers.org/rec/BER IPA-10

Berner, Eta (ed.). 2007. *Clinical Decision Support Systems.* New York: Springer.

Brennan, Cathy A. et al. 2003. "Management of Diagnostic Uncertainty in Children with Possible Meningitis: A Qualitative Study." *British Journal of General Practice* 53: 626–631.

Broadbent, Alex. 2019. *Philosophy of Medicine.* New York: Oxford University Press.

Burger, Edward B. and Michael Starbird. 2005. *Coincidences, Chaos, and All That Math Jazz: Making Light of Weighty Ideas.* New York: W.W. Norton and Company.

Caldaria, Antonio et al. 2020. "COVID-19 and SARS: Differences and Similarities." *Dermatologic Therapy* 33 (4): e13395. https://doi.org/10.1111/dth.13395

Caliendo, Angela M., and Kimberly E. Hanson. 2022. "COVID-19: Diagnosis." *UpToDate.* August 15. www.uptodate.com/contents/covid-19-diagnosis?search= COVID-19%20Diagnosis&source=search_result&selectedTitle=1~150&usa ge_type=default&display_rank=1

Centers for Disease Control and Prevention. 2021a. "COVID-19 Data Tracker." August 14. https://covid.cdc.gov/covid-data-tracker/#datatracker-home

Centers for Disease Control and Prevention. 2021b. "COVID-19 Symptoms." May 11. www.cdc.gov/coronavirus/2019-ncov/symptoms-testing/symptoms.html

Centers for Disease Control and Prevention. 2021c. "COVID-19 Vaccinations." April 16. www.cdc.gov/vaccines/covid-19/index.html

Centers for Disease Control and Prevention. 2021d. "Estimated COVID-19 Burden." August 29. www.cdc.gov/coronavirus/2019-ncov/cases-updates/bur den.html

Centers for Disease Control and Prevention. 2021e. "Health Equity Considerations and Racial and Ethnic Minority Groups." May 11. www.cdc.gov/coronavirus/ 2019-ncov/community/health-equity/race-ethnicity.html

Centers for Disease Control and Prevention. 2022a. "COVID-19 Data Tracker." August 14. https://covid.cdc.gov/covid-data-tracker/#datatracker-home

Centers for Disease Control and Prevention. 2022b. "How to Protect Yourselves and Others." August 11. www.cdc.gov/coronavirus/2019-ncov/prevent-getting-sick/prevention.html

Centers for Disease Control and Prevention. 2022c. "Long COVID or Post-COVID Conditions." September 1. www.cdc.gov/coronavirus/2019-ncov/long-term-effects/index.html

Centers for Disease Control and Prevention. 2022d. "Symptoms of COVID-19." March 22. www.cdc,gov/coronavirus/2019-ncov/symptoms-testing/sympt oms.html

Chang, Chiang-Hua et al. 2023. "Nursing Home to Nursing Home Transfers during the Early COVID-19 Pandemic." *Journal of the American Medical* Directors Association 24 (4) (April): 441–446. doi:10.1016/j.jamda.2023.01.028. Epub 2023 Feb 10. PMID: 36878263; PMCID: PMC9915045.

Chen, Ray Ming. 2020. "Randomness for Nucleotide Sequences of SARS-CoV-2 and Its Related Subfamilies." *Computational and Mathematical Methods in Medicine* (November 14): 8819942. doi:10.1155/2020/8819942. PMID: 33273962; PMCID: PMC7683162.

Cohen, Pieter, and Kelly Gebo. 2022. "COVID-19: Management of Adults with Acute Illness in the Outpatient Setting." *UpToDate*. August 1. www.uptodate.com/contents/covid-19-evaluation-of-adults-with-acute-illness-in-the-outpatient-setting?search=COVID-19%20Treatment&source=search_result&selectedTitle=1~150&usage_type=default&display_rank=15

The Commonwealth Fund. 2021. "Understanding and Ameliorating Medical Mistrust Among Black Americans." January 14. www.commonwealthfund.org/publications/newsletter-article/2021/jan/medical-mistrust-among-black-americans

The Conversation Project. 2022. "Helping People Share Their Wishes for Care through the End of Life." https://theconversationproject.org/wp-content/uploads/2020/04/tcpcovid19guide.pdf

"Coronavirus History." 2020. "Coronavirus History." May 13. www.webmd.com/lung/coronavirus-history

Cotofan, Maria et al. 2021. "Work and Well-Being During COVID-19: Impact, Inequalities, Resilience, and the Future of Work." *World Happiness Report 2021*. https://worldhappiness.report/ed/2021/work-and-well-being-during-covid-19-impact-inequalities-resilience-and-the-future-of-work

Crenshaw, Kimberlé Williams. 1989. "Demarginalizing the Intersection of Race and Sex: A Black Feminist Critique of Antidiscrimination Doctrine, Feminist Theory, and Antiracist Politics." *University of Chicago Legal Forum* 14: 538–554.

Crenshaw, Kimberlé Williams. 1991. "Mapping the Margins: Intersectionality, Identity Politics, and Violence Against Women of Color." *Stanford Law Review* 43: 1241–1299

Cutter, Mary Ann G. 2003. *Reframing Disease Contextually*. Dordrecht, The Netherlands: Kluwer Academic Publishers.

Cutter, Mary Ann G. 2012. *The Ethics of Gender-Specific Disease*. New York: Routledge.

Cutter, Mary Ann G. 2018. *Thinking Through Breast Cancer: A Philosophical Exploration of Diagnosis, Treatment, and Survival*. New York: Oxford University Press.

Davis, Kathy. 2008. "Intersectionality as Buzzword: A Sociology of Science Perspective on What Makes a Feminist Theory Successful." *Feminist Theory* 9: 67–85.

Deville, Jaime G. et al. 2022. "COVID-19: Management in Children." *UpToDate*. August 15. www.uptodate.com/contents/covid-19-management-in-children?search=COVID-19%20Treatment&source=search_result&selectedTitle=3~150&usage_type=default&display_rank=3

Djulbegovic, Benjamin. 2021. "Ethics of Uncertainty." *Patient Education and Counseling* 104 (11) (November): 2628–2634.

Domen, Ronald E. 2016. "The Ethics of Ambiguity: Rethinking the Role and Importance of Uncertainty in Medical Education and Practice." *Academic Pathology* 16 (June): 1–7.

Dorn, Stan, and Rebecca Gordon. 2021. "The Catastrophic Cost of Uninsurance: COVID-19 Cases and Deaths Closely Tied to America's Health Coverage Gaps." *Families USA: The Voice for Health Care Consumers*. March

4. https://familiesusa.org/resources/the-catastrophic-cost-of-uninsurance-covid-19-cases-and-deaths-closely-tied-to-americas-health-coverage-gaps/

Douedi, Steven, and Jeffrey Miskoff, J. 2020. "Novel Coronavirus 2019 (COVID-19): A Case Report and Review of Treatments." *Medicine (Baltimore)* 99: e20207. https://doi.org/10.1097/MD.0000000000020207

Dunlop, Mark, and Richard M. Schwartzstein. 2020. "Reducing Diagnostic Error in the Intensive Care Unit. Engaging Uncertainty When Teaching Clinical Reasoning." *ATS Scholar* 1: 364–371.

Eddy, David M. 1984. "Variations in Physician Practice: The Role of Uncertainty." *Health Affairs* 3 (2): 74–89.

Ellsberg, Daniel. 1961. "Risk, Ambiguity, and the Savage Axioms." *Quarterly Journal of Economics* 75: 643–649.

Engebretsen, Eivind et al. 2016. "Uncertainty and Objectivity in Clinical Decision Making: A Clinical Case in Emergency Medicine." *Medicine, Health Care, and Philosophy* 19: 595–603.

Engel, George. 1980. "The Clinical Application of the Biopsychosocial Model." *The American Journal of Psychiatry* 137 (5): 535–544.

Engel, George. 1981. "The Need for a New Medical Model: A Challenge for Biomedicine." In *Concepts of Health and Disease: Interdisciplinary Perspectives.* Edited by A.L. Caplan et al., 589–607. Boston: Addison-Wesley.

Engelhardt, H. Tristram, Jr. 1996. *Foundations of Bioethics.* 2nd ed. New York: Oxford University Press.

Feinstein, Alvan R. 1967. *Clinical Judgement.* New York: The Williams and Wilkins Company.

Foucault, Michel. 1973 [1963]. *Birth of the Clinic: An Archeology of Medical Perception*, translated by A.M. Sheridan Smith. New York: Pantheon Books.

Fourie, Carina. 2013. "Moral Distress and Moral Conflict in Clinical Ethics." *Bioethics* 29 (2): 91–97.

Fourie, Carina. 2017. "Who Is Experiencing What Kind of Moral Distress? Distinctions for Moving from a Narrow to a Broad Definition of Moral Distress." *AMA Journal of Ethics* 19 (6): 578–584. https://journalofethics.ama-assn.org/article/who-experiencing-what-kind-moral-distress-distinctions-moving-narrow-broad-definition-moral-distress/2017-06

Fox, Renée C. 1980. "The Evolution of Medical Uncertainty." *Milbank Memorial Fund* 58: 2–49.

Foxwell, Anessa M. 2022. "Dying in Isolation." In *Nurses and COVID-19: Ethical Considerations in Pandemic Care.* Edited by C.M. Ulrich and C. Grady, 19–33. Cham, Switzerland: Springer.

Freed, Meredith et al. 2022. "Deaths Among Older Adults Due to COVID-19 Jumped During the Summer of 2022 Before Falling Somewhat in September." *KFF.* October 6. www.kff.org/coronavirus-covid-19/issue-brief/deaths-among-older-adults-due-to-covid-19-jumped-during-the-summer-of-2022-before-falling-somewhat-in-september

Gan, Connie C.R. et al. 2020. "Acrylic Window as Physical Barrier for Personal Protective Equipment (PPE) Conservation." *American Journal of Emergency Medicine* 38 (7): 1532–1534.

Gigerenzer, Gerd. 2002. *Calculated Risks: How to Know When Numbers Deceive You*. New York: Simon and Schuster.

Gold, Joshua I, and Michael N. Shadlen. 2007. "The Neural Basis of Decision Making." *Annual Review of Neuroscience* 30: 535–574.

Gordon, Deb. 2022. "Amid Healthcare's Great Resignation, Burned Out Workers Are Pursing Flexibility and Passion. *Forbes*. May 17. www.forbes.com/sites/debgordon/2022/05/17/amid-healthcares-great-resignation-burned-out-workers-are-pursuing-flexibility-and-passion/?sh=12e52a0b7fda

Gordon, Michael R., and Warren P. Strobel. 2023. "A Lab Leak in China Most Likely Origin of COVID Pandemic." *Wall Street Journal*. February 26. www.wsj.com/articles/covid-origin-china-lab-leak-807b7b0

Gøtzsche, Peter C., and Henrik R. Wulff. 2007. *Rational Diagnosis and Treatment: Evidence-based Clinical Decision-making*. 4th ed. West Sussex, England: John Wiley & Sons.

Grady, Christine. 2022. "The Emotional and Moral Remnants of COVID-19: Burnout, Moral Distress, and Mental Health Concerns." In *Nurses and COVID-19: Ethical Considerations in Pandemic Care*. Edited by C.M. Ulrich and C. Grady, 53–62. Switzerland: Springer.

Greenhalgh, Trisha. 2021. "Moral Uncertainty: A Case Study of COVID-19." *Patient Education and Counseling* 104: 2643–2647.

Groopman, Jerome. 2007. *How Doctors Think*. Boston, Massachusetts: Houghton Mifflin Company.

Han, Paul K.J. 2021. *Uncertainty in Medicine: A Framework for Tolerance*. New York: Oxford University Press.

Han, Paul K.J. et al. 2011. "Varieties of Uncertainty in Health Care: A Conceptual Taxonomy." *Medical Decision Making* 6(November–December): 828–838.

Han, Paul K.J. et al. 2017. "A Taxonomy of Medical Uncertainties in Clinical Genome Sequencing." *Genetic Medicine* 19(August 19): 918–925.

Han, Paul K.J. et al. 2019. "Uncertainty in Health Care: Towards a More Systematic Program of Research." *Patient Education and Counseling* 102(10): 1756–1766. doi:10.1016/j.pec.2019.06.012

Hansson, Sven Ove. 2013. *The Ethics of Risk: Ethical Analysis in an Uncertain World*. Switzerland: Springer.

Henry, Tanya Allbert. 2022. "Medicine's Great Resignation?" *AMA*. January 18. www.ama-assn.org/practice-management/physician-health/medicine-s-great-resignation-1-5-doctors-plan-exit-2-years

Higgins-Dunn, Noah. 2020. " 'You Are Not Listening,' Fauci Tells Sen. Rand Paul During a Senate Hearing on the Coronavirus." *CNBC.com*. September 23 www.cnbc.com/2020/09/23/you-are-not-listening-fauci-tells-rand-paul-during-senate-hearing.html

Higgins-Dunn, Noah. 2021. "COVID Was the Third Leading Cause of Death Among Americans in 2020, Behind Heart Disease and Cancer, CDC Says." *CNBC.com*. March 31. www.cnbc.com/2021/03/31/covid-was-third-leading-cause-of-death-in-us-in-2020-behind-heart-disease-and-cancer-cdc-says.html

Hill, Latoya, and Samantha Artiga. 2022. "COVID-19 Cases and Deaths by Race/Ethnicity: Current Data and Changes Over Time." *KFF*. August 22.

www.kff.org/coronavirus-covid-19/issue-brief/covid-19-cases-and-deaths-by-race-ethnicity-current-data-and-changes-over-time

Ho, Anita. 2020. "Western Arrogance in the Face of COVID." *iainews* 87 (April 8). https://iai.tv/articles/western-arrogance-in-the-face-of-covid-19-auid-1401

Honigsbaum, Mark. 2019. *The Pandemic Century: One Hundred Years of Panic, Hysteria and Hubris.* New York: W.W. Norton and Company.

Hunink, M.G. Myriam. et al., 2014. *Decision Making in Health and Medicine.* 2nd ed. Cambridge, England: Cambridge University Press.

Hutto, Emily. 2022. "'Of' or 'With' COVID? Pandemic Deaths Are Getting Harder to Count." *Medscapes.* November 11, medpagetoday.com.

Jackson, Griffin Paul. 2020. "Hospital Restrictions Bar Chaplains from Ministering Bedside." *Christianity Today.* March 25. www.christianitytoday.com/news/2020/march/chaplain-ministry-hospital-restrictions-covid-19-us.html

Jameton, Andrew. 1984. *Nursing Practice: Ethical Issues.* Hoboken, New Jersey: Prentice-Hall.

Jameton, Andrew. 2017. "What Moral Distress in Nursing History Could Suggest about the Future of Health Care." *AMA Journal of Ethics* 19 (6): 617–628.

Johnson, L. Syd M. 2021. *The Ethics of Uncertainty: Entangled Ethical and Epistemic Roots in Disorders of Consciousness.* New York: Oxford University Press.

Kahneman, Daniel. 2011. *Thinking, Fast and Slow.* New York: Farrar, Straus, and Giroux.

Kahneman, Daniel et al. 1982. *Judgment Under Uncertainty: Heuristics and Biases.* New York: Cambridge University Press.

Kant, Immanuel. 1985 [1785]. *Foundations of the Metaphysics of Morals.* Translated by L.W. Beck. New York: Macmillan.

Kasper, Jürgen et al. 2008. "Decision-Related Uncertainties Perceived by People with Cancer-Modelling the Subject of Shared Decision Making." *Psychooncology* 17 (1) (January): 42–48.

Katz, Jay. 1984. "Why Doctors Don't Disclose Uncertainty." *The Hastings Center Report* 14 (1): 35–44.

Kayser, Joshua et al. 2021. "Managing Moral Distress During a Pandemic." *Society of Critical Care Medicine Blog.* December 21. www.sccm.org/Blog/December-2021/Managing-Moral-Distress-During-a-Pandemic

Kim, Arthur Y., and Rajesh T. Ghandi. 2022. "COVID-19: Management in Hospitalized Adults." *UpToDate.* August 15. www.uptodate.com/contents/covid-19-management-in-hospitalized-adults?search=COVID-19%20Treatment&source=search_result&selectedTitle=2~150&usage_type=default&display_rank=2

Koffmann, Jonathan et al. 2020. "Uncertainty and COVID-19: How Are We To Respond?" *Journal of the Royal Society of Medicine* 113 (6) (June): 211–216

Leap, Edwin. 2023. "Removing the COVID Blindfold: A Few Lessons Learned as We Move Beyond the Public Health Emergency." *Rural Rx.* May 10 www.medpagetoday.com/opinion/rural/104441

Lei, Ruipeng, and Renzong Qiu. 2020. "Chinese Bioethicists: Silencing Doctor Impeded Early Control of Coronavirus." *Global Health, Hastings Bioethics*

Forum. February 13. www.thehastingscenter.org/coronavirus-doctor-whistl eblower/

Linzer, Mark et al. 2022. "Responding to the Great Resignation: Detoxify and Rebuild the Culture." *Journal of General Internal Medicine* 37 (16) (December): 4276–4277. doi:10.1007/s11606-022-07703-1. Epub 2022 Jun 29. PMID: 35768678; PMCID: PMC9243774.

Lowrey, Annie. 2021. "Growing Old, Alone." *Atlantic.* February 2 www.thea tlantic.com/ideas/archive/2021/01/social-depression-America-failed-its-elderly/ 617496

Maestripieri, Lara. 2021. "The COVID-19 Pandemics: Why Intersectionality Matters." *Frontiers in Sociology* 6 (Article 642662). www.frontiersin.org/artic les/10.3389/fsoc.2021.642662/full

Mandavilli, Apoorva. 2021. "The U.S. Is Getting a Crash Course on Scientific Uncertainty." *New York Times.* 8/23/21. www.nytimes.com/2021/08/22/health/ coronavirus-covid-usa.html

Marcum, James A. 2008. *An Introductory Philosophy of Medicine.* Dordrecht, The Netherlands: Springer.

McDaniel, Rueben R., and Driebe, Dean J. 2001. "Complexity Science and Health Care Management." *Advances in Health Care Management* (*Advances in Health Care Management, Vol. 2*), 11–36. Bingley: Emerald Group Publishing Limited. https://doi.org/10.1016/S1474-8231(01)02021-3

Mill, John Stuart. 1979 [1861]. *Utilitarianism.* Edited with an introduction by G. Sher. Indianapolis, Indiana: Hackett Publishing Company.

Mishel, Merle H. 1981. "The Measurement of Uncertainty in Illness." *Nursing Research* 30 (5) (September–October): 258–263.

Mishel, Merle H. 1988. "Uncertainty in Illness." *Journal of Nursing Scholarship* 20: 225–232.

Mol, Annemarie. 2002. *The Body Multiple: Ontology in Medical Practice.* Durham, North Carolina: Duke University Press.

Murthy, Vivek. 2022. "Confronting Healthcare Worker Burnout and Well-Being." *New England Journal of Medicine* 387: 577–579.

National Catholic Bioethics Center. 2021. "Vaccine Exemption Template Letter." *Bi-Weekly Newsletter.* July 7. www.ncbcenter.org/ncb-news/vaccineletter

National Consumer Voice for Quality Long-Term Care. 2021. "Statement on the New York Attorney General's Report on the Effects of COVID-19 on Nursing Homes in New York." *Newsletter.* February 5. https://theconsumervoice.org/iss ues/other-issues-and-resources/covid-19

National Human Genome Research Institute. 2023. "Personalized Medicine." August 25. www.genome.gov/genetics-glossary/Personalized-Medicine

Neilson, Susie. 2020. "A Year of the Pandemic, in 26 photos." *Business Insider.* December 23. www.businessinsider.com/coronavirus-pandemic-in-pho tos-one-year-2020-12

Nelson-Becker, Holly, and Christina Victor. 2020. "Dying Alone and Lonely Dying: Medica Discourse and Pandemic Conditions." *Journal of Aging Studies* 55(September 23): 100878–100888. https://pubmed.ncbi.nlm.nih.gov/ 33272449

Noddings, Nel. 1984. *Caring: A Feminine Approach to Ethics and Moral Education*. Oakland, California: University of California Press.

Nussbaum, Martha. 2003. *Upheavals of Thought: The Intelligence of Emotions*. Cambridge, England: Cambridge University Press.

Oxford English Dictionary. 1994. *Uncertainty*. Oxford, England: Oxford University Press.

Pathman, Donald E. et al. 2022. "Moral Distress Among Clinicians Working in US Safety Net Practices During the COVID-19 Pandemic: A Mixed Methods Study." *British Medical Journal Open* 12 (8): e061369. doi:10.1136/bmjopen-2022-061369. PMID: 36008061; PMCID: PMC9421917.

Pellegrino, Edmund D. 2008. *A Philosophy of Medicine Reborn*. Notre Dame, Indiana: Notre Dame University Press.

Pence, Gregory E. 2021. *Pandemic Bioethics*. Peterborough, Ontario: Broadview Press.

"Pictures of the Year: COVID." 2021. Reuters. December 9. www.reuters.com/news/picture/pictures-of-the-year-covid-idUSRTXLAJS8

"Pierre de Fermet Mathematician." 2021. *The Story of Mathematics* www.storyof mathematics.com/17th_fermat.html

Pomare, Chiara et al. 2019. "A Revised Model of Uncertainty in Complex Healthcare Settings: A Scoping Review." *Journal of Evaluation in Clinical Practice* 25: 176–1782.

Preeti, R. John et al. 2021. "Ethical Considerations for a COVID-19 Vaccine Mandate." *Critical Connections Blog. Society for Critical Care Medicine*. June 17. www.sccm.org/Blog/June-2021/Ethical-Considerations-for-a-COVID-19-Vaccine-Mand

Rawls, John. 1971. *A Theory of Justice*. Cambridge, Massachusetts: Cambridge University Press.

Reznek, Lawrie. 1987. *The Nature of Disease*. London: Routledge and Keegan Paul.

Rosén, Mans et al. 2022. "The One-Sided Explanations of a Multifactorial Coronavirus Disease." *Scandinavian Journal of Public Health* 50 (1): 19–21. doi:10.1177/14034948211026540

Roy, Avrik. 2020. "Nursing Home Deaths From COVID-19: U.S. Historical Data." *freopp.org*. July 15. https://freopp.org/nursing-home-deaths-from-covid-19-u-s-historical-data-b4ad44cfc48e

Ruble, Eric. 2021. "State Shutting Down Never-Used Colorado Convention Center as Emergency Hospital." *KDVR.com*. January 19. https://kdvr.com/news/coronavirus/state-shutting-down-never-used-colorado-convention-center-as-emergency-hospital

Rueda, Jon. 2021. "Ageism in the COVID-19 Pandemic: Age-Base Discrimination in Triage Decisions and Beyond." *History and Philosophy of the Life Sciences* 43 (3): 91. doi:10.1007/s40656-021-00441-3. PMID: 34258692; PMCID: PMC8276843.

Rushton, Cynda Hylton. 2016. "Moral Resilience: A Capacity for Navigating Moral Distress in Critical Care." *AACN Advanced Critical Care* 27 (1): 111–119. https://aacnjournals.org/aacnacconline/article/27/1/111/2285/Moral-Resilience-A-Capacity-for-Navigating-Moral

Rushton, Cynda Hylton. 2017. "Cultivating Moral Resilience." *American Journal of Nursing* 117 (2) (February): S11–S15. https://pubmed.ncbi.nlm.nih.gov/28085701/

Rushton, Cynda Hylton. 2018. *Moral Resilience: Transforming Moral Suffering in Healthcare.* New York: Oxford University Press.

Rushton, Cynda Hylton, and Kathleen Turner. 2020. "Suspending our Agenda: Considering What Will Serve When Confronting Moral Challenges." *AACN Advanced Critical Care* 31 (1): 98–105. https://pubmed.ncbi.nlm.nih.gov/32168521

Santhosh, Lekshmi et al. 2019. "Diagnostic Uncertainty: From Education to Communication." *Diagnosis* 6: 121–126.

Sapkota, Nabin et al. 2021. "The Chaotic Behavior of the Spread of Infection During the COVID-19 Pandemic in the United States and Globally." *IEEE Access* 9: 80692–80702. www.ncbi.nlm.nih.gov/pmc/articles/PMC8545195

Sasser, Jade S. et al. 2021. "Commentary: Intersectional Perspectives on COVID-19 Exposure." *Journal of Exposure Science and Environmental Epidemiology* 31: 401–403.

Sassower, Raphael, and Mary Ann G. Cutter. 2007. *Ethical Choices in Contemporary Medicine.* Stocksfield, England: Acumen.

Sassower, Raphael, and Michael Grodin. 1987. "Scientific Uncertainty and Medical Responsibility." *Theoretical Medicine* 8: 221–234.

Sauvages de la Croix, Francois Bossier de. 1768. *Nosologia Methodica Sistens Morborum Classes Juxta Sydenhami Mentem et Botanicorum Ordinem,* 5 Vols. Montpellier, France: Fratrum de Tournes.

Schleicher, Gunter K. et al. 2020. "Case Study: A Patient with Asthma, Covid-19 Pneumonia and Cytokine Release Syndrome Treated with Corticosteroids and Tocilizumab." *Wits Journal of Clinical Medicine* 2 (SI) (April): 47–52. doi:10.18772/26180197.2020.v2nSIa9

Sepielli, Andrew. 2009. "What to Do When You Don't Know What to Do." *Oxford Studies in Metaethics* 4: 5–28.

Sherwin, Susan. 2006. "Personalizing the Political." In *The Voice of Breast Cancer in Medicine and Bioethics.* Edited by M. Rawlinson and S. Lundeed, 3–19. Cham, Switzerland: Springer.

Simpkin, Arabella L., and Richard M. Schwatzstein. 2016. "Tolerating Uncertainty—The Next Medical Revolution." *The New England Journal of Medicine* 3 (November): 1713–1715.

Sopory, Pradeep et al. 2019. "Communicating Uncertainty During Public Health Emergency Events: A Systematic Review." *Review of Communication Research* 7: 67–108.

Sox, Harold C. et al. 2013. *Medical Decision Making.* 2nd ed. Oxford, England: Wiley-Blackwell.

Stegenga, Jacob. 2018. *Care and Cure: An Introduction to Philosophy of Medicine.* Chicago, Illinois: University of Chicago Press.

Sylvester, Shirley V. et al. 2022. "Sex Differences in Sequelae from COVID-19 Infection and in Long COVID Syndrome: A Review." *Current Medical Research and Opinion.* 38(June 20): 1391–1399. https://pubmed.ncbi.nlm.nih.gov/35726132

Tannert, Christof et al. 2007. "The Ethics of Uncertainty." *EMBO Reports* 8 (10): 885–974.

Thagard, Paul. 2021. "The Ethics of Mandatory Vaccination." *Psychology Today*. April 26. www.psychologytoday.com/us/blog/hot-thought/202104/the-ethics-mandatory-vaccination

Thompson, R. Paul., and Ross Upshur. 2017. *Philosophy of Medicine: An Introduction*. New York: Routledge.

Timmer, John. 2020. "SARS-CoV-2 Looks Like a Hybrid of Viruses from Two Different Species." *Arstechnica*. June 1. https://arstechnica.com/science/2020/06/sars-cov-2-looks-like-a-hybrid-of-viruses-from-two-different-species

Todhunter, Isaac. 1865. *A History of the Mathematical Theory of Probability, From the Time of Pascal to that of Laplace*. Cambridge: Macmillan and Co.

Tuana, Nancy. 2006. "The Spectrum of Ignorance: The Women's Health Movement and Epistemologies of Ignorance." *Hypatia* 21 (3): 1–19.

U.S. Department of Health and Human Services. 2023. "Fact Sheet: COVID-19 Public Health Emergency Transition Roadmap." February 9. www.hhs.gov/about/news/2023/02/09/fact-sheet-covid-19-public-health-emergency-transition-road map.html#:~:text=Based%20on%20current%20COVID%2D19,day%20on%20May%2011%2C%202023

U.S. Food and Drug Administration. 2021a. "Emergency Use Authorization for Vaccines to Prevent COVID-19." February. www.fda.gov/regulatory-informat ion/search-fda-guidance-documents/emergency-use-authorization-vaccines-prev ent-covid-19

U.S Food and Drug Administration. 2021b. "FDA and CDC Lift Recommended Pause on Johnson & Johnson (Janssen) COVID-19 Vaccine Use Following Thorough Safety Review." April 23. www.fda.gov/news-events/press-announ cements/fda-and-cdc-lift-recommended-pause-johnson-johnson-janssen-covid-19-vaccine-use-following-thorough

Ulrich, Connie M., and Christine Grady. 2019. "Moral Distress and Moral Strength Among Clinicians in Health Care Systems: A Call for Research." *NAM Perspective*. Washington, DC: National Academy of Medicine.

Vordermark II, Jonathan S. 2019. *An Introduction to Medical Decision-Making: Practical Insights and Approaches*. Cham, Switzerland: Springer.

Wehner, Peter. 2021. "NIH Director: We Need an Investigation into the Wuhan Lab-Leal Theory." *The Atlantic*. June 2. www.theatlantic.com/ideas/archive/2021/06/francis-collins-nih/619065/

Wolpaw, Terry et al. 2009. "Using SNAPPS to Facilitate the Expression of Clinical Reasoning and Uncertainties: A Randomized Comparison Group Trial." *Academic Medicine* 84: 517–524.

Woolever, Donald R. 2008. "The Art and Science of Clinical Decision Making." *Family Practice Management* 15 (5) (May): 31–36. www.aafp.org/fpm/2008/0500/p31.html

World Health Organization. 2020. "Naming the Coronavirus Disease (COVID-19) and the Virus that Causes It." September 9. www.who.int/emergencies/disea ses/novel-coronavirus-2019/technical-guidance/naming-the-coronavirus-dise ase-(covid-2019)-and-the-virus-that-causes-it

World Health Organization. 2021. "WHO Coronavirus (COVID-19) Dashboard." August 14. https://covid19.who.int

World Health Organization. 2022. "Tracking SARS-CoV-2 Variants." June 14. www.who.int/activities/tracking-SARS-CoV-2variants

Wulff, Henrik R. 1981. *Rational Diagnosis and Treatment: An Introduction to Clinical Decision-Making.* 2nd ed. Oxford, England: Blackwell Scientific Publications.

Wulff, Henrik R. et al. 1986. *Philosophy of Medicine.* Oxford, England: Blackwell Scientific Publications.

Zhou, Amy et al. 2021. "Is Precision Medicine Relevant in the Age of COVID-19?" *Genetic Medicine* 23: 999–1000. https://doi.org/10.1038/s41436-020-01088-4

Glossary of Terms in Biomedical Ethics

ambiguity: inexactness, the quality of being open to more than one interpretation.

autonomy: ethical duty to respect self-determination. Autonomy involves two conditions: (1) liberty, or independence of controlling influences, and (2) agency, capacity for intentional action.

axiology: the philosophical study of value.

beneficence: ethical duty to benefit another. Entails various kinds of duties, such as the protection and defense of the rights of others, the prevention of harm from occurring to others, the removal of conditions that will cause harm to others, help for persons with disabilities, and the rescue of persons who are in danger.

bioethics/biomedical ethics: the study of ethical issues in biomedicine.

care ethics/the ethics of care: care ethics focuses on duties to maintain human relationships by contextualizing and promoting the well-being of care-givers and care-receivers within social systems of power. Special attention is given to acts of compassion for the vulnerable, or those most dependent on others.

certainty: a state of being reliably true or clear.

clinical decision-making: a cognitive process based on known best practices (based on evidence and research), awareness of current clinical problem, and knowledge of the patient.

clinical problem: a general term that includes disease, illness, deformity, and dysfunction.

compassion: a state of sympathy for another, and especially the vulnerable, and taking actions to assist

complexity: a state or quality of having any different parts connected or related to each other.

constructivism: the view that knowledge and reality are constructed as opposed to discovered.

dignity: a state of being worthy of respect by the self or others.

empiricism: the view that knowledge is derived from sense perception.

epistemic: of or relating to knowledge or knowing.

epistemology: the philosophical study of knowledge.

equity: the quality or state of fairness.

ethics: the philosophical study of good and bad, and right and wrong, as these judgments have to do with the actions and character of individuals, families, communities, institutions, and societies, and global orders.

fact: an empirically verifiable statement that correlates with an object or state of affairs that exists.

feminist philosophy: a term for a wide range of host of positions and approaches that focus on the need for accounts of reality, knowledge, and values that respond to the plights or oppression of marginalized and oppressed persons.

health equity: a state in which everyone has a fair opportunity to attain their optimal health regardless of identities of difference (e.g., gender, race, economic class, age, and disability).

informed consent: in medicine, the moral and legal process of obtaining permission from a patient before a medical intervention occurs. Involves that the patient is competent, relevant medical information and options are disclosed, and that the patient understands what is being agreed to.

integrative: that which is brought together or incorporated into a whole. In medicine, refers to medicine that combines evidence-based medicine with alternative approaches in health care.

intersectionalism: in philosophy and sociology, refers to a way of thinking and practice that situates how systems of inequity based on identities of difference (e.g., sex/gender, race/ethnicity, ability/disability, class/economic status, religion/spirituality, age) intersect and interact to create dynamics (e.g., of power) and experiences (e.g., of oppression) that define experience.

issue of uncertainty: a topic or problem regarding uncertainty.

justice: ethical duty to achieve equity.

locus of uncertainty: location or stakeholder of uncertainty.

metaphysics: the philosophical study of that which is beyond the physical.

moral distress: a state of feeling unable to carry out a morally appropriate ethical action. Can lead to a variety of responses, such as moral fatigue, moral injury, moral betrayal, moral guilt, moral suffering, moral overload, moral resignation, moral burnout, and moral nihilism.

moral resilience: the capacity of an individual to sustain or restore moral integrity in response to moral complexity, confusion, fear, distress, or setbacks.

moral value: a claim of worth or praiseworthiness.

nonmaleficence: ethical duty to minimize or avoid harm. Entails various kinds of duties, such as avoiding harm, minimizing harm, or preventing harm.

normative ethics: the philosophical study in ethics concerned with criteria of what is morally good or bad, or right or wrong. Focuses on "what *ought* to be done."

objectivity: the state of being independent of mind. Usually contrasts with subjectivity.

ontology: the philosophical study of being.

practical ethics: the philosophical study in ethics concerned with what ought to be done in a situation. Entails a focus on ethical case analysis.

probability: the extent to which some thing or event is likely to occur.

rationalism: the philosophical view that knowledge is derived from reason.

realism: the philosophical view that there is a reality to be discovered and not simply constructed.

reflective equilibrium: a state of balance or coherence among a set of values arrived at by deliberative mutual adjustment among moral appeals.

right: in moral philosophy, a claim or entitlement to be treated a certain way because of one's status (e.g., autonomy, dignity).

risk: the relation of benefit to burden, harm, or cost.

risk assessment: a calculation of benefit over burden, harm, or cost. A measure of the likelihood of an adverse effect.

source of uncertainty: the root of something or way of thinking.

subjectivity: the state or quality of originating from one's mind or being influenced by personal feelings or opinions.

uncertainty: a conscious recognition of doubt, lack of clarity, confusion, or suspicion.

value: as a noun, a sign of worth or assessment of comparison. As a verb, to assign worth to something or someone.

welfare: best interest or well-being.

Index

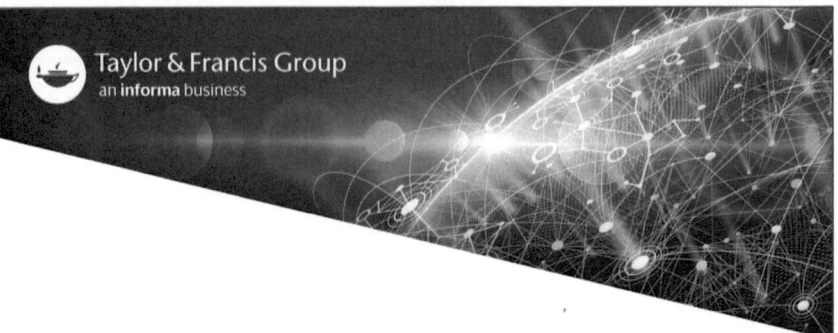
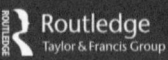
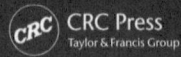